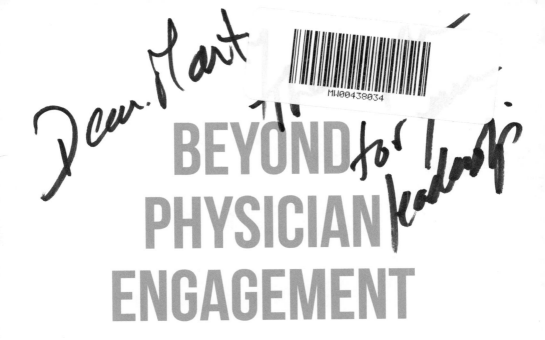

BEYOND PHYSICIAN ENGAGEMENT

A ROADMAP TO PARTNER WITH PHYSICIANS TO BE

ALL IN

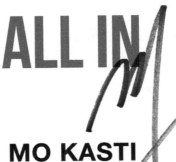

MO KASTI

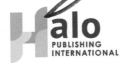

Halo
PUBLISHING
INTERNATIONAL

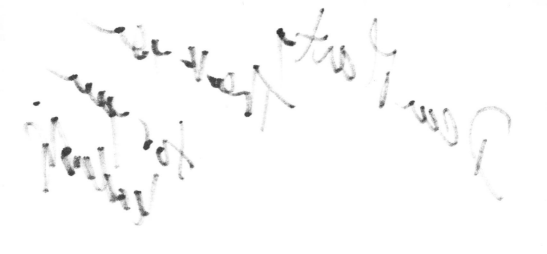

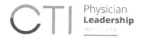

CTI | Physician **Leadership** INSTITUTE

ISBN: 978-1-61244-645-5
Library of Congress Control Number: 2018913563

Printed in the United States of America

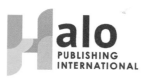

Halo Publishing International
1100 NW Loop 410
Suite 700 - 176
San Antonio, Texas 78213
1-877-705-9647
www.halopublishing.com
contact@halopublishing.com

To all the physicians we have had the privilege to work with over the years and their noble mission of saving lives and helping humanity.

To all the healthcare leaders that have had the courage to go beyond engagement and truly partner with their physicians and team members.

To my wife, the love of my life, Rana for her support, encouragement, and dedication to our family, healthcare, and CTI.

To my two emerging leaders, Adam and Jude: you inspire me and keep me young and grounded.

To my mom, dad, and siblings who showed me what love is.

Table of Contents

Foreword

From the moment I met Mo Kasti and selected him from 16,000 applications to be part of my MG100 Pay it Forward coaching initiative, I realized that his passion for healthcare was palpable. I knew from his resume and his work that he was a primary authority on physician leadership, strategy and innovation and that he gets into the trenches with the leaders of healthcare systems, large and small to help them transform healthcare. I knew he was willing to get his hands dirty, but I didn't fully understand why until I got to know more about his incredible life story.

Growing up in war-torn Lebanon in the late 70s, Mo volunteered as a young man to help others including rescuing dozens of families from the rubble. He watched physicians, with few resources, work tirelessly to save lives - including his own uncle and father.

He later came to America, the wealthiest country in the world, where in 1999, the Institute of Medicine published a report called, "Do No Harm" in which it was estimated that 100,000 people in the U.S. die needlessly from preventable medical errors each year – more than those who died in the Lebanese civil war.

This report was a fuel to Mo's passion and launched his life's work in healthcare transformation.

His enthusiasm for that mission has not wavered over the years. On any given day, you can find him coaching physicians and leaders, vigorously sketching strategy maps on whiteboards, scribbling innovative ideas on lunch napkins, and traveling the globe to capture the pain points of doctors, nurses, C-suite administration and patients.

Mo is ALL IN, and now I understand why.

In this book, Mo has cracked the code on physician engagement. **The evidence is clear, increased engagement leads to better clinical outcomes.** Weaving together the art of leadership, neuroscience, and communication, Mo has created a methodology that, if adopted, could quite literally save lives.

Too often we try to measure engagement the way we measure other metrics – as a cost, as a managerial responsibility or as a means to an end. But engagement, as Mo explains, is none of these things. It is a two-way commitment between professionals. It is situational and ever-changing. To put it plainly – it cannot simply be crossed off a to-do list.

The beauty of this book is in the way Mo has woven the intangible state of engagement (as Dr. Ron Paulus describes, 'I know it when I see it') with tangible tools for achieving it.

If you need inspiration, there are several case studies in the book that showcase what can happen when engagement efforts succeed.

Going beyond the traditional definition of engagement takes work. If you're ready to take your organization to the next level, I encourage you to commit. Channel your inner med-school student, get out your highlighter, and deep-dive into this book.

For Mo, it's clear this book is the result of a very personal journey.

I invite you to join him on his journey. May this roadmap be your guide and serve as your inspiration toward a better healthcare system for us all.

Life is good.

Marshall

Marshall Goldsmith is the New York Times #1 bestselling author of "Triggers", "Mojo", and "What Got You Here Won't Get You There".

Introduction

Google the word "engagement" and gold and diamonds will fill your screen with links to:

- Engagement rings and diamond wedding rings | Tiffany & Co.

- Find the perfect diamond engagement rings...

- The strange (and formerly sexist) economics of engagement ring...

and

- 10 things no one tells you about shopping for an engagement ring...

But modify your search to find "physician engagement" and you may find yourself singing the *Wedding Bell Blues*.

Physician engagement, after all, isn't achieved by simply buying a ring and expecting physicians to say "I do." It's a lot more complicated and difficult to do.

There are hundreds of books that have been written on engagement, yet engagement is at an all-time low, especially among physicians – a mere 10 percent. Recent Gallup Organization studies of more than 6,000 physicians in the U.S. found that only 10 percent were fully engaged with their hospitals, while 42 percent were actively disengaged. All of these books fall short when it comes to explaining physician engagement. I believe we have approached engagement the wrong way in healthcare. We've made it a metric and held our managers accountable. **Physicians are professionals and don't need to be parented. They need to be partnered with.**

This book is about speaking the truth as professionals. It puts the accountability on both parties to act as partners to co-lead, co-create, and make the *choice* to be engaged or not.

I've seen the power of strong physician engagement firsthand. I've also witnessed the problems that occur when physicians are not engaged. It isn't pretty. It is a safety threat.

In my previous book: **Physician Leadership: The Rx for Healthcare Transformation**, I made the case for physician leadership leading the healthcare transformation and provided a roadmap for transformational leadership which included leading with purpose, leading with strategy, leading self, engaging others, and leading for results.

This book outlines a progressive roadmap that blends the art of leadership, neuroscience, language, and conversation acts. It is a roadmap that enables both professional parties to go beyond engagement and to establish, or re-establish, trust through smart conversations and small sprints.

It is time to go beyond engagement.

In this book, I'll take a look at all aspects of engagement and give you step-by-step advice on ways to improve engagement, especially among physicians and other members of the healthcare team. I will also share stories and examples of leaders who have been successful at engaging their physicians in strategy as well as clinical operations.

Engagement is critical in today's ever-changing healthcare. Achieving strong engagement:

- Reduces burnout

- Improves clinical outcomes

- Boosts patient experience scores

- Helps guarantee better patient safety

- Promotes a positive culture throughout the organization

- Leads to more satisfied staff and reduces turnover

- Increases productivity

- Results in a patient-centric, value-based environment that is crucial for the future of healthcare

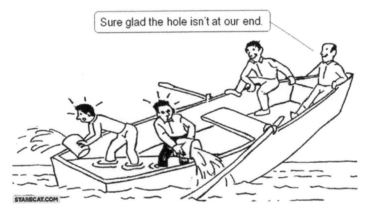

If you think all that sounds too good to be true, don't take my word for it. Look at what other industries outside of healthcare are saying about the absolute need for engaged employees.

Why Engagement?

"Engagement is a top talent issue facing organizations today," states the Deloitte consulting firm on its website. "Building an environment that is fulfilling, meaningful, and fun is not only good for employees, but can also potentially result in better business outcomes, including higher productivity, increased efficiency, higher levels of customer satisfaction, and better overall business results."

"Creating a positive culture of high employee engagement will not only help your employees but also your business", states the Society of Human Resource Management Foundation. "In fact, the evidence is clear: employees who are engaged in their work and committed to their organizations give companies crucial competitive advantages, including higher productivity and lower employee turnover," the organization states in an executive briefing statement (*SHRM*).

In his days at General Electric, CEO Jack Welch, "cited employee engagement as the most crucial measure of a company's health—more important than customer satisfaction or cash flow. Engaged employees will 'go the extra mile' to serve customers and to be an advocate for the organization. Focus on increasing employee engagement first, and customer satisfaction and bottom line results will follow." (*SHRM*)

Physicians and researchers interviewed for this book who have studied, taught, and published articles about engagement for years are quick to concur. "It's all about culture, and when you improve the culture, people are happier. There's more productivity and more life," said Alan Rosenstein, MD, MBA, a practicing internist at ValleyCare in San Francisco, California, and longtime behavioral management consultant. "And they're less likely to leave."

Rosenstein asserts that engaged workers want to be proud of what they do; they want to contribute to their company's success and feel that the job they do and their opinions matter.

Sam Bahreini, founder and COO of the retail analytics firm, VoloForce, echoes that viewpoint in an October 2015 article for *Entrepreneur* entitled "Employee Engagement is More Important Than the Customer" (*Bahreini-2015*). "Problems don't begin with customers," Bahreini explains. "They start with you and your employees. When customers expect a fantastic experience but receive a third-rate one, you can lose them forever." He emphasized that, "You need to be your own customer."

William (Marty) Martin, Psy.D., a licensed clinical psychologist, writer, and speaker who has conducted in-depth research into human behavior, said that being a satisfied employee isn't enough. Employees can be satisfied, but not truly engaged. "Engagement is a step above satisfaction."

Research by the National Business Research Institute, a firm with more than 30 years of experience conducting scientific, psychological research for businesses, found that only one out of three employees is truly engaged (*Infographic -NBRI*).

THE VALUE OF EFFECTIVE ENGAGEMENT

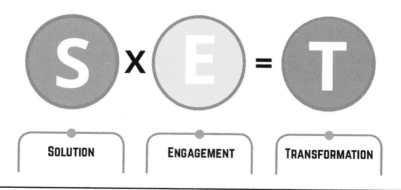

| SOLUTION | ENGAGEMENT | TRANSFORMATION |

I believe that engagement, especially physician engagement, is an essential factor in healthcare transformation. It has a multiplier effect! Engaging physicians and staff is essential to sustainable success and transformation.

Engagement is completely off for a majority of U.S. workers, according to statistics compiled by Gallup. They found that slightly more than 50 percent of employees were "not engaged," and 17 percent were "actively disengaged." (*Adkins-2016*)

On a global level, Gallup data reported in 2017, a staggering 87 percent of employees around the world were not engaged.

GALLUP'S THREE TYPES OF EMPLOYEES

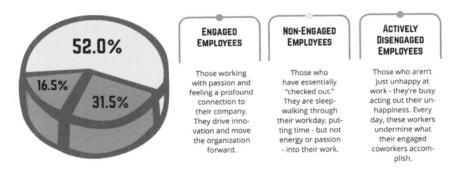

	ENGAGED EMPLOYEES	**NON-ENGAGED EMPLOYEES**	**ACTIVELY DISENGAGED EMPLOYEES**
52.0% / 16.5% / 31.5%	Those working with passion and feeling a profound connection to their company. They drive innovation and move the organization forward.	Those who have essentially "checked out." They are sleep-walking through their workday, putting time - but not energy or passion - into their work.	Those who aren't just unhappy at work - they're busy acting out their unhappiness. Every day, these workers undermine what their engaged coworkers accomplish.

What is the actively disengaged employee doing? They are not just unhappy at work; they are busy acting out their unhappiness. Every day, these workers undermine what their engaged coworkers accomplish. Engaged employees, on the other hand, are involved, enthusiastic and committed to their work. Gallup's extensive research shows that employee engagement is strongly connected to business outcomes essential to an organization's financial success, such as productivity, profitability, and customer engagement. Engaged employees support the innovation, growth, and revenue that their companies need.

For those companies that understand and actively pursue an engaged workforce, the payoff is big. Gallup reported that organizations with highly engaged workforces outperform their peers by a whopping 147 percent in earnings per share.

Disengaged employees aren't bad employees. They just do the minimum amount of work required to keep the job, according to Gallup. Sound familiar?

So what exactly is engagement? There are loads of definitions out there, many of them quite similar.

What is Engagement?

There are many definitions of Engagement. One definition involves a promise and a commitment-like promise to marry. Another definition involves conflict, like engaging the enemy. Here are a few more:

"Engagement is the extent to which someone feels passionate about his or her job, is committed to the organization, and puts discretionary effort into his or her work." (*CustomInsight*)

"Engagement is the emotional commitment the employee has to the organization and its goals." (Kruse-2012)

"Physician engagement is an intangible process that depends on the degree to which doctors are proud, loyal, and committed to a hospital's mission, vision, and values," said Tom Atchison in "Leading Healthcare Cultures: How Human Capital Drives Financial Performance."

However, engagement should not be confused with happiness or satisfaction. Think of it this way: two friends can be happy and satisfied with their friendship, but not be engaged to be married. Engagement in the workplace, just as it is for couples considering marriage, is a much deeper commitment.

What is the Origin of Employee Engagement Concept?

The roots of engagement lie historically in the survival of human species where early humans needed the engagement of their fellow tribesmen to hunt, protect their lives, and expand their influence over other tribes. However, the term employee engagement is a recent concept. The first use of the term employee engagement occurred in a 1990 Academy of Management Journal by William A. Kahn. Kahn's article on the psychological conditions of personal engagement and disengagement at work examined the conditions which contribute to this phenomenon. He discovered that the individual and contextual sources of meaningfulness, safety, and availability had a significant impact on engagement. In the 2000s, engagement gathered speed, depth, and breadth. Google searches of the term in the early 2000s offered about 50,000 results and now the same search term offers 47,500,000 results. Tweets on employee engagement would appear about every 30 minutes five years ago and now occur just about every minute.

As the global marketplace grew larger, workers became more mobile in their jobs, according to an article published by *HRZone* in November 2013 (*O'byrne-2013*). Prior to the global expansion, workers tended to take a job and stay with it for many years, perhaps staying at the same company for their entire work life.

Think about American automobile manufacturing as an example. Workers would land a job at a production facility, and while they may have switched positions or been promoted within the company, they stayed with the manufacturer for

30 or 40 years, retiring with a nice pension. You can also be sure that they drove one of the automobiles produced by their company for all those years as a sign of deep loyalty to the employer. With the influx of production of foreign cars in the U.S. in the 1980s and 90s, the days of working for one company for years on end began to wane.

Employee loyalty was refocused and workers had more options. They were mobile, and their loyalties became more self-serving. They had valuable skills and could work for the highest bidder; they slowly became free of their employers and realized they were empowered to go elsewhere with their skills. Of course, other factors were at work, too. The U.S. economy was becoming less industrial and more service-oriented. Eventually, the information age would arrive and the freedom to work anywhere, anytime, from a computer became reality. But there was a problem.

Employers who once counted on loyal workers sticking around for years were experiencing a brain-drain of sorts. They were losing some of their best workers to competitors, and it costs much more to replace a worker who leaves than to retain a skilled, reliable employee. So what's the best way to retain and keep those valuable employees motivated? In his book "Drive," Daniel Pink explored what motivated people in life and in work. His findings were fascinating. He quoted a study by MIT, University of Chicago and Carnegie Mellon. The study demonstrated that incentive and better pay did not always result in better performance or retention. As long as the task involved used only mechanical skill, bonuses worked as expected, but once the task called for rudimentary cognitive skill, larger rewards actually led to poorer performance and less loyalty. Pink found that there are three factors that lead to better engagement, performance, and personal satisfaction: autonomy, mastery, and purpose. Autonomy is the desire to be self-directed. Pink asserts that traditional management techniques lead to compliance, but if you want engagement allow autonomy and self-direction. Mastery is the urge to get better at certain tasks, and purpose gives meaning and sense of value that attracts better talent and engagement.

In the current age, engagement has become essential in performance, transformation, and change management. To improve performance, accelerate change, and/or increase the prospect of success, we need to engage people. We must positively influence and encourage others. Only then can we hope to achieve a specific goal faster, better, and more efficiently.

In healthcare, change and transformation have become constant. The industry is having a hard time adapting to the new world of health, value, and consumerism. The odds of succeeding are not very promising. After all, statistics show that 70 percent of change efforts fail and one key factor contributing to the high failure rate is the lack of engagement and buy-in. We are seeing a high rate of stress and burnout due to lack of adaptability. We are reminded by Deming that if people don't adapt their thinking and actions to the change, they are doomed to becoming irrelevant: "It is not the strongest or smartest species that survive, it is the most adaptable to change."

How is Physician Engagement Measured? Or is it Measured?
Lack of consistent definition and measurement

There is no consistent agreement on how physician engagement is defined and how it is measured. When you look at the questions of various common instruments like Gallop, IBM, and the Advisory Board, you have to wonder what is being measured. Are we measuring happiness, communication, confidence, pride, passion, integrity, alignment, control, allegiance, economic alignment, loyalty, autonomy, or interest in physician leadership?

For example, Gallup uses the following statements as indicators of physician engagement:

- I trust the hospital or health system's leadership team.

- I am involved in making decisions about clinical policy at my hospital/health system.

- I am involved in making decisions about administrative policy at my hospital or health system.

- My hospital/health system has been successful at navigating the economic, technological, and regulatory changes taking place in healthcare today.

- My hospital/health system has been proactive in dealing with changes in healthcare brought about by the Affordable Care Act.

- Time is made available for me to pursue clinical, academic, and/or research projects in which I am interested.

- I have control over my own schedule.

- I am satisfied with the quality of communication across the hospital or health system.

- I have the staffing and support I need to do my job well.

- I am satisfied with my level of work/life balance.

- There are programs in place at my hospital/health system that promote physicians' health and well-being.

On the other hand, the Advisory Board defines engagement in terms of the following twelve "drivers": [21]

1. I would recommend this organization to a friend or relative to receive care.

2. The actions of this organization's executive team reflect the goals and priorities of participating clinicians.

3. This organization supports my professional development.

4. This organization is open and responsive to my input.

5. This organization provides excellent service to patients.

6. I am interested in physician leadership opportunities at this organization.

7. This organization is well prepared to meet the challenges of the next decade.

8. Over the past year I have not been asked by this organization to do anything that would compromise my values.

9. This organization provides excellent clinical care to patients.

10. This organization supports the economic growth and success of my individual practice.

11. This organization supports my desired work-life balance.

12. I have the right amount of autonomy in managing my individual practice.

The advisory board scores engagement in other instruments and studies through the answers to four questions:

1. What is your willingness to go above and beyond?

2. What is your level of loyalty to the organization?

3. Would you recommend the organization to others as a good place to work?

4. Do you see yourself at the organization in the next few years?

Needless to say, the lack of consistency in definition and measurement is a challenge in itself and contributes to difficulty of impacting physician engagement in healthcare.

I Know it When I See it

Dr. Ron Paulus, CEO of Mission Health believes that engagement metrics are not reflective of what is going on in the trenches. They are a snapshot in time that may change depending on context. A clinician may care about something today and be fully engaged, but may not engage in another issue that he or she doesn't care about. Does that mean they are not engaged?

Dr. Paulus describes engagement as follows: "With engagement, it is not an absolute metric. It is about trends. I look for global trends with groups and individuals. Are we improving over time?

At Mission, our weekly Standout Check-Ins are level one of our engagement approach. As leaders, are we engaging our team members by replying to their weekly check-ins? Our team members start the conversation with: 'Here is what I need from my team leader.' By responding to that need, you can drive accountability and, ultimately, engagement."

Paulus said he also can detect engagement by watching others. "Simply put, I know engagement when I see it in a room or in a meeting. I watch the interactions between people and watch for body language. Are people leaning into the conversation, building on each other's thoughts, and having a constructive conversation? Are they additive to one another or is the conversation dominated by only a few? Is there a high level of stress in the room?"

New Definition of Engagement

I offer the following engagement definition:

Engagement is a two-way emotional commitment between professionals to fulfill on a specific mission or task. Engagement is situational and changes over time. It is a choice we make based on what we care about in the moment or in the future. It is a muscle that needs to be exercised over time.

WHAT IS ENGAGEMENT

WHAT ENGAGEMENT IS:	WHAT ENGAGEMENT IS NOT:
• Situational or situation-driven	• One Size Fits All
• A Two-Way Commitment	• One-Way Commitment (Manager)
• A Choice	• A Metric
• Intentional	• A Favor
• Changes Over Time	• An End
• Investment	• A Cost
• Emotional	• Logic-Based
• A Source of Energy	• A Draining Activity
• A muscle	• Happiness or Satisfaction
• Part of Being a Professional	

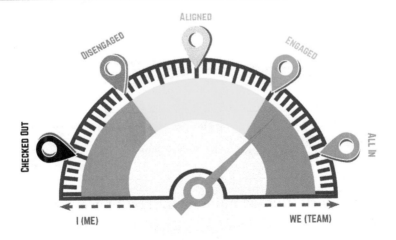

In addition, I believe engagement is a continuum of commitment that ranges from being ALL IN to being ALL OUT. There are three distinct ranges or zones:

1. RED ZONE: Starts from being Disengaged to ALL checked OUT. In the Red Zone, people are focused on themselves or their needs and are demonstrating their opposition actively or passively.

2. YELLOW ZONE: From being Disengaged to Engaged. In the Yellow Zone, we observe alignment to a shared purpose, goals, and priorities. Both sides are acting in a supportive way to drive better outcomes.

3. GREEN ZONE: From Engaged to ALL IN. In the green zone engagement goes a step further. It's about being fully invested and energized to the point that the person is proactively **putting in discretionary effort**. People in the green zone are fully vested, proactive, have a sense of urgency, and are able to rally others.

UNDERSTANDING THE ZONES

ZONE	RED ZONE	YELLOW ZONE	GREEN ZONE
DESCRIPTION	Actively disengaged	Share organizational or team purpose and goals	Actively engaged, energized and act as an owner
FOCUS	Me	I and we	We
ENERGY	Passive aggressive to actively disruptive	Neutral	Active, Proactive, Intentional
ACTIONS & BEHAVIORS	Acting, deciding and behaving in ways that support self-interest Us versus them	Acting, deciding, and behaving in ways that support the organizational purpose Satisfied with the status quo	Seeing engagement as part of the profession Has a bias for action, is optimistic, triggers to the best in others, actively involved and/or involve others ALL IN
KEY INDICATORS	I don't trust the others or the organization's leadership I am not proud to say I practice here	I know the purpose and the goals of the organization I trust the leadership I am willing to engage	I am proud to say I practice here I feel a sense of ownership I am willing to recommend this organization to my colleagues

Martin supports this continuum by pointing out that there may well be different levels of engagement depending on an individual's likes and dislikes.

For example, one employee may be totally engaged when meeting and greeting customers on the floor of a retail store, but ask them to spend the day restocking supplies in the warehouse that's adjacent to the store, and they may plod through the task showing little or no engagement.

Martin also noted that people may have different reasons for getting engaged in their work. Some may be seeking self-satisfaction, others may be working to support the greater good of the company, while others may be highly engaged in order to get a raise or promotion to a new position. Think of a musician who wants to improve his skills on his instrument. The musician is engaged and contributes to the improved performance of the orchestra, but the engagement is totally centered on the musician's need to improve himself. He may not really be thinking at all about the overall performance of the orchestra.

"I think there are multiple paths to engagement, not just one path," Martin said. He cautioned that it's important not to try to gauge engagement on extraneous factors or individual actions. "Me taking all my vacation days doesn't mean I'm more engaged or less engaged. Me going to lunch or taking two 15-minute breaks doesn't mean I'm more or less engaged. The indicators to high engagement are high contribution, high performance, and high satisfaction."

Employment Does not Equal Engagement

When it comes to engagement, it's important to note that employment does not mean engagement. Merely providing a paycheck, insurance benefits, and vacation and sick leave does little to encourage or ensure engagement.

Martin noted that this idea was first outlined by psychologist Frederick Herzberg and his two-factor theory. The theory states that there are factors in the workplace that can lead to satisfaction and some that can sow the seeds of dissatisfaction.

The two-factor theory distinguishes between "hygiene factors," such as a decent salary, good benefits, and job security, and "motivational factors," such as playing a role in making decisions, having the chance to do work that's meaningful, and being recognized for a job well-done.

Companies—particularly senior leaders—must do much more than simply provide hygiene factors in order to achieve engagement. Just as the wedding ring is only a symbol of engagement, employers shouldn't think engagement can be bought by just supplying additional perks. That's not to say perks and rewards aren't important. They are. True engagement, however, is much deeper.

Martin said perks, in some ways, actually may be detrimental to engagement. How could that happen? Take, for example, a company that provides employees with free food, child care, and maybe even an errand service to try to engage employees. What they may end up with, Martin explained, is an expectation that employees work a 60- or 70-hour work week. The idea is that the company is offering all the perks in order to give the employees more time—to work. "I guess you could call it 'perk enslavement,'" Martin said.

So how are non-clinical organizations and some of the most highly recognized companies in the country successfully engaging employees? Let's take a look.

One Size Does Not Fit All

The most important rule to remember is that one size doesn't fit all employees or companies.

Gary Ridge CEO of WD-40 Company, the manufacturer of WD-40 lubricant, has been able to achieve, in 2018, 93% engagement among his employees.

Gary believes: "Purpose-driven, passionate people guided by their values create amazing outcomes."

Gary spends a considerable among of his time ensuring alignment between organizational values and employees needs and values. Gary emphasizes that one size does not fit all as demonstrated by the relationship between the level of engagement and individual's hierarchy of needs (using Maslow's Hierarchy of Needs).

MASLOW'S HIERARCHY OF NEEDS APPLIED TO EMPLOYEE ENGAGEMENT

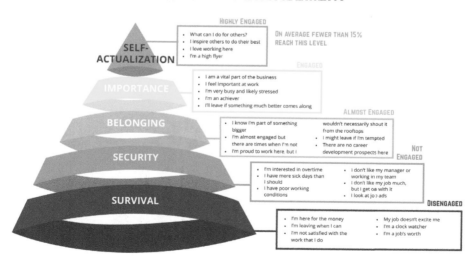

A January 2017 article in *Harvard Business Review* identified four retailers that were among the best places to work in the U.S. (*Ton and Kalloch-2017*). As we all know, retail can be one of the most grueling industries to be working in. Long hours, low pay, and dealing with unhappy customers face-to-face can certainly take a toll on employees. But places like HEB, Costco, Trader Joe's, and Quiktrip rose to the top of the retail engagement surveys by creating cultures where employees are challenged, yet happy, and appear to thrive.

The *HBR* authors interviewed leaders in each company, and here's a sampling of what they said:

Craig Boyan, HEB's president and COO, "likens his company's culture to a favorite teacher—not necessarily the nicest but the one that set the bar high and pushes you to do better than you ever thought you could." The company gives pay incentives each year and challenges employees in all parts of the company to come up with innovative ways to show they deserve the raises.

Costco takes a similar approach, the article states, setting the bar high for employees, paying them well, and encouraging them to take ownership of their work. One employee, a butcher, rose through the ranks to become a meat manager who helps open new stores.

Doug Rauch, former Trader Joe's president, sounded a similar refrain, and talked to *HBR* about the importance of empowering employees to do what's right for customers and for the company. "Having employees' voices matter," he said, "it is important to keeping them engaged."

Likewise, an article in *Forbes* described the very different ways that large and well-known companies are engaging employees, and much of it comes down to figuring out what truly makes the employees happy and eager to do a good job (*Vorhauser-Smith-2013*).

Recreational Equipment (REI) deeply connects with employees on social media and holds what it calls "camp fires" that allow employees to participate in discussions and debates. According to the *Forbes* article, more than 4,500 of REI's 11,000 employees had logged in to the camp fire site in its first year.

Other top-rated companies, such as Google, combine open communication and a fun atmosphere along with some unusual perks such as free gourmet food and an on-site laundry, the article stated. At top-rated SAP Software Corporation, extraordinary efforts are made to make sure employees understand their jobs and honest, open communication is encouraged throughout the company, with leaders actually listening and responding to employee ideas, the *Forbes* article stated.

That's one I've seen many times at CTI. When senior leaders are transparent and actively listening to their employees and physicians' concerns and responding in very human terms, engagement tends to be high.

The opposite is true as well. In companies where the CEO and senior leaders cloister themselves off from the rest of the employees, and decisions are handed down without employee input—and often come as unexpected surprises—engagement is in the tank.

"The most important things are trust and respect," Rosenstein agreed. But it doesn't only apply to senior leaders. Middle managers also must have the skills and techniques to encourage engagement among their direct reports.

Timothy J. Keogh, PhD, a communications expert who has studied engagement and workplace behaviors and taught at

Tulane University in New Orleans, Louisiana, and The Citadel in Charleston, South Carolina, said in an interview that many of the problems with lack of engagement actually stem from supervisors and the annual performance evaluations.

"The performance evaluation is done by a supervisor or manager, and managers hate to do them, so what they do is manage the event. The managers talk 80 percent of the time and that is exactly the wrong thing to do to engage an employee," Keogh explained.

He said managers should let the employees do more than 80 percent of the talking. The employees want to be heard; they want to know someone is listening to them. Keogh also said the evaluations end up being a bust, and the employee would return to his or her workspace less engaged than when they left, if the manager shows little or no interest in their ideas, concerns, and desires.

"A fundamental part of being engaged in an organization is having a superior listen to you. And what's the number one complaint we hear when we talk to a disgruntled employee?" Keogh asked. It's "no one listens to me!"

At WD-10, Gary Ridge encourages employee engagement by promoting a culture of learning. He calls them Learning Moments: "We don't make mistakes, we have learning moments" he said.

Why is Physician Engagement Important?

The terrain of healthcare is changing and is proving to be somehow inhospitable these days. Healthcare is going through a transformation similar to the disruption other industries experienced moving from the craft age to the industrial age, and again from the industrial age to today's information age. However, the speed of this healthcare transformation has been accelerated to transition from a volume- based to a value-based care. To be successful at this exponential transformational rate requires that all key stakeholders specially physicians to be actively engaged.

HEALTHCARE IS FINALLY GOING THROUGH ITS TRANSFORMATION

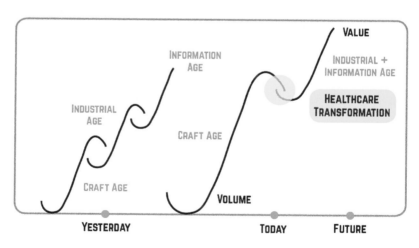

Rosenstein, at Valley Health in San Francisco, considers engagement to be especially important in healthcare organizations. "Engagement is critical in healthcare. You're talking about people's health or sometimes life and death situations. Health and well-being are more important than building a better computer, so having an engaged clinical workforce is something healthcare organizations should strive for."

It gets a much more complicated because engagement involves many different players in the healthcare arena. "It is a multidisciplinary type of approach. It's all the physicians, clinical workers, patients, and the patients' families. Then you also have to consider the individual patient and their values," Rosenstein said.

As the healthcare financial model moves from volume-based to value-based reimbursement, engagement takes on an even larger role. Patient experience scores and positive outcomes matter. High scores are worth money, and an engaged healthcare workforce leads to a better work environment, more satisfied patients, and better outcomes.

There is proof emerging that an engaged healthcare workforce improves outcomes, quality of care, and patient satisfaction. "As Towers Watson's research with clients shows, when hospitals create an engaging and high-performance-oriented work experience, they not only improve patient satisfaction, but also quality of care outcomes," stated an October 2013 article in *Harvard Business Review* (*Sherwood-2013*). The same Towers Watson's study found that less than half of the U.S. hospital workforce was highly engaged.

A study by Gallup and Loma Linda University Medical Center in California support these findings. "When healthcare employees work in a safe environment and are engaged, the chances are much greater that they will perform activities that are known drivers of better patient safety outcomes," a Gallup article about the study stated (*Burger and Sutton-2014*).

Physician Engagement has direct impact on the revenue, growth and the bottom line. Gallup found that physicians who were partially or fully engaged were 26% more productive than physicians who were not engaged or actively disengaged. This increase equates to an average of $460,000 in patient revenue per physician per year. In other words, a health system could improve its bottom line by nearly half a million dollars a year each time it successfully engages one of its less engaged physicians.[20] When comparing this system's physician engagement data with referral volume, Gallup found that fully engaged physicians gave the hospital an average of 3% more outpatient referrals and 51% more inpatient referrals than physicians who were not engaged or actively disengaged.

Jackson Healthcare's 2016 physician engagement survey results mirrored Gallup's results – more engaged physicians are more productive and have greater loyalty to the organization.[22]

Where is Physician Engagement Today?

Various studies paint a dim picture of engagement in healthcare.

Recent Gallup Organization studies of more than 6,000 physicians in the U.S. found that only 10 percent are fully engaged with their hospitals, while 42 percent are actively disengaged.

Data compiled by the Advisory Board for 2015 through 2016 showed physician engagement at about 35 percent, while engagement among other healthcare workers was about 40 percent, according to Sarah Rothenberger, managing director of Survey Solutions at the organization.

"Employee engagement from 2015 to 2016 saw a slight uptick, but physician engagement has remained relatively flat," she said.

The organization surveyed hundreds of thousands of healthcare employees and scored engagement primarily through the answers to four questions:

1. What is your willingness to go above and beyond?

2. What is your level of loyalty to the organization?

3. Would you recommend the organization to others as a good place to work?

4. Do you see yourself at the organization in the next few years?

"What we're really getting at is whether the employee is emotionally committed to the role and emotionally committed to the organization itself."

Rothenberger said the Advisory Board sees engagement as a driver of better outcomes, too. "We do see a connection between engagement and patient satisfaction. Engaged employees are much more likely to be rated as higher performers. We see less turnover at highly engaged organizations. We also see organizations with high levels of engagement have high patient safety scores."

Advisory Board data over the years showed that the greatest drivers of physician engagement remain relatively constant. "Responsiveness to physician input and executive actions reflective of physician priorities are consistently among the highest impact drivers of engagement for economic affiliates, surpassing even care quality and support for economic growth," a report from the group stated.

Excellent service, which wasn't ranked in the Advisory Board survey in 2015, made a great leap forward in importance in 2016. "This organization provides excellent service to patients" now rates as one of the strongest drivers of engagement for the overall medical staff, including physicians, the survey found.

A deeper look into some of the data collected and shared by Rothenberger uncovered some interesting insights:

- Engagement among employed physicians actually has stalled in the last year, but engagement among independent physicians at the health systems where they work is slightly higher.

- Generational differences may impact engagement in many industries, but among physicians, it remains a factor with only slight variations among young doctors and older.

- Although it's not necessarily clear why some physician specialties see higher rates of engagement than others, the Advisory Board data found that among the most highly engaged and aligned specialties included infectious disease, pathology, oncology/hematology, plastic surgery, vascular surgery, pulmonology/critical care, and hospitalists. Among those with lower levels of engagement were allergy/immunology, dermatology, gastroenterology, orthopedic surgery, urological surgery, and vascular surgery.

The physicians and researchers we interviewed agreed that engaged physicians play a crucial part in spreading engagement throughout the medical staff. One poorly behaving, disgruntled, or disengaged physician can cast a pall on all those with whom he or she works. By contrast, a thoroughly engaged physician can lift the spirits and attitudes of the rest of the medical staff, setting a positive example of engagement that spreads to others.

After all, most physicians pursue medicine as a life calling because they want to do something positive and worthwhile, care for people, and heal those who are suffering. "I think for those workers that choose the healthcare profession initially, engagement comes easier," Martin said. "They are choosing to serve the sick, serve the infirm, and serve the disabled. That's their motivation going in; that's how they're socialized."

Martin suspects that physician engagement is highest when doctors first leave residency and begin the actual practice of medicine. They would have spent many years of their lives preparing for that moment, and they finally have the skills and degrees needed to care for patients on their own. Then reality hits.

Medical records must be completed rapidly and accurately. Evidence-based protocols are dictated and must be followed. The volume of patients to be seen each day continually rises. Non-clinical administrators may question a physician's care delivery and expenses. Insurance companies intervene with more questions and more paperwork. "Then what I think happens is, over the course of bad experiences, lack of time, lack of feedback, and perhaps being socialized by negative, cynical people, all of that chips away at their engagement," Martin said. As a result, their satisfaction and willingness to contribute start to dissolve.

When Martin works with burned out physicians and nurses, he often asks them why they chose to go to medical school or nursing school. "Inevitably, their story is full of altruism, higher purpose, and flow." But then when he asks about the working conditions they are currently facing, the stories lose their altruism and focus on obstacles that have little or nothing to do with direct patient care.

Rosenstein has seen the same thing. "Other forces begin to interfere with what they want to do," he said. "They feel they're losing their autonomy and losing control of the situation. And they feel they're being told something by someone who doesn't understand clinical medicine. Time spent on administrative issues, medical records, and all this stuff is being thrust on them and that's not what they signed on for."

Keogh, from The Citadel, agreed. "Physicians don't often see the bigger picture. They are very patient-centric. Trying to get a doc to see the organizational goals can be difficult." And if physicians or other healthcare workers sense that an organization is more about money than patient care, engagement easily can decline.

"Healthcare is very hierarchical, very command and control. It's very status and privilege-oriented, and what also happens is once you get in it, you realize the patient isn't necessarily first. Whoever is saving money or bringing in money, they're first," Martin said. "So for physicians, they ask: 'Why be engaged with an organization that's all about the money?' Because that's just antithetical to their values."

Why Physician Engagement is Different and More Difficult To Achieve?

Why is it more difficult to achieve physician engagement in healthcare than in other industries? Why is physician engagement different than employee engagement? Great questions. No easy answers.

William Cors, MD, MMM, FACPE, Vice President and Chief Medical Officer at Lehigh Valley Health Network's Lehigh Valley Hospital in Pennsylvania, said in an interview that it often takes quite a bit of work to engage physicians.

"There is no secret sauce to achieving engagement for physicians. And engagement doesn't guarantee you'll get the desired clinical outcomes, but it may help."

Physician Engagement is easier to pronounce than to achieve for many reasons which I have grouped in five areas:

1. **System and Process**

2. **Purpose**

3. **Leadership**

4. **Interpersonal or Culture**

5. **Personal**

ENGAGEMENT FACTORS

LEADERSHIP
- Lack of Clinical Leadership
- Lack of Onboarding

SELF/PERSON
- Retirement
- Lack of Energy/Time
- Stress/Burnout

PURPOSE
- Alignment

SYSTEM
- Lack of Focus (LOS)
- Hassle Factors
- Complexity
- Lack of Innovation

CULTURE
- Lack of Trust
- Generational Differences
- Lack of Psychological Safety

System and Process Factors

Hassle Factor Index™

Amazon has effectively transformed our online shopping habits, and that is causing the bankruptcy of many stores such as Sears and Kmart. Amazon has been able to achieve dominance and secure our loyalty by being maniacal about shopper experience by laser focusing on the hassle factors and friction points in every step of our shopping journey, from the time we are thinking of buying something to the time we decide to return it. With all this advancement of our understanding of decreasing hassle factors and points of complexity in work systems in general, it is unfortunate that the complexity of healthcare has gone up.

This increased complexity has become an invisible source of stressors that only physicians and healthcare workers face and that exacerbate the trend toward burnout.

In a recent study conducted by CTI's Physician Leadership Institute, we asked physicians to identify the hassle factors that contribute to stress, frustration, and potentially disengagement.

Hassle Factor Themes

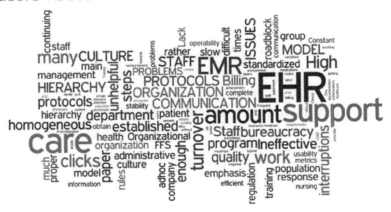

The daily grind of seeing patient after patient, the threat of lawsuits, regulations, documentation and billing, quality metrics, and dashboards were among those mentioned.

The five major sources of hassle were:

1. The Electronic Health Records (EHR) system. Documentation and Pajama time

2. Cultural challenges such as not having effective collaboration with peers and lack of communication

3. Lack of/poor clinical leadership that is an effective voice/representation

4. Increased focus on financial and productivity

5. Increased complexity of organization

Reducing hassle factors is part of a three-legged strategy at Mission Health as well as a way to send a message of care to the providers. Ron Paulus, CEO describes it as follow "We call it reNEW. How do you take the inefficiency out of the system and out of people's way so they can practice and deliver the best possible and safest care? By focusing on the system and system processes, we are sending a message to our staff and providers that we care about them and we understand the complexity of our systems and that they are not perfect. Although we may not be able to solve everything, especially when it comes to regulatory-induced hassles, trying to fix systems and processes shows that you care and makes life better."

Do you have a way to measure and remove hassle factors for your providers? Do you know your customers, physicians and employees' Hassle Factor Index?

Purpose Factors

In his book *Drive: The Surprising Truth About What Motivates Us*, Daniel Pink documented that professionals are motivated intrinsically in three different ways: autonomy, mastery, and purpose (*Pink-2012,*). In healthcare, while patient care is a unifying purpose, we have been seeing more and more divergence in alignment of purpose between the physicians and the organizations they work with leading to lack of engagement.

1. Renter versus Owner

Historically, physicians were independent of the hospital or health system and spent time at the hospitals admitting their patients and/or performing a procedure. They engaged with the hospital out of care for the patients and the community. There was a sense of common purpose and they acted as co-owners. As financial incentives and reimbursement changed over time and hospitals started hiring their own providers, physicians found themselves in competition with the hospital - driving their engagement way down. They became renters.

2. Going to the Dark Side

Aligning oneself to the goals of the organization remains a huge challenge when doctors who get engaged are regarded as "sellouts" or labeled as having "gone to the dark side".

3. Independence and Autonomy

The number of physicians in the United States grew 150 percent between 1975 and 2010, roughly keeping with population growth, while the number of healthcare administrators increased 3,200 percent for the same time period.

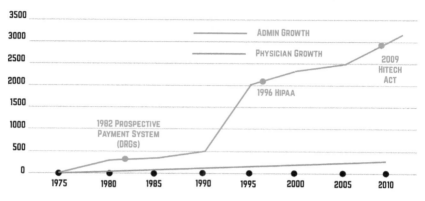

With more people trying to manage their care, physicians have felt a loss of autonomy over decisions as simple as setting their schedules. The historical divide of medical staff independence and hospital/organization is still in existence. There is a need for bridging the divide by focusing on a common purpose – patient care.

Cultural Factors

There are many cultural factors that lead to lack of engagement and those include conflicting cultures, lack of trust, and generational differences.

1. Lack of alignment between "expert culture" and "collective culture"

What people don't realize is that the vast differences between collective and expert cultures lead to tension, conflict, disengagement, and stress, especially if the physician and the hospital lack alignment around purpose.

Most healthcare professionals and administrators are acclimated to a collective culture, whereas physicians belong to an expert culture. In the former category are such professionals as nurses, therapists, administrators, and support staff. These professionals usually work in groups, tend to avoid conflict, and are not high risk-takers. Physicians, in contrast, tend to be individualistic risk-takers who prize their autonomy. Outside of patient care, they are more likely to be motivated by self-interest than by group values.

Physicians and administrators also may differ in their perception of teamwork. As Joe Bujak wrote in "Inside the Physician Mind: Finding Common Ground with Doctors," "physicians view themselves as members of an expert culture who conceive of teams in terms of individual performance, like members of a golf team who compete in their own matches. However, administrators tend to see themselves as part of an interdependent affiliated culture, like members of a volleyball team, who dig, set, and spike to win points".

2. Lack of Trust

The relationship between physicians and administrators has become tense, challenged, and fractured - talking over one another rather than to each other.

While one explanation is that *change is hard*—and the healthcare industry is changing more rapidly than anyone is able to keep up with – there is another explanation. The groups don't understand or trust one another.

3. Generational Differences

Younger physicians have different values than baby boomer physicians. Many of them would rather spend time with friends and family than sit through another meeting.

At Mission Health, Ron Paulus is improving engagement, especially physician engagement, by focusing on the cultural factors. The Mission Health team is creating a strength-based culture that leverages the physician's unique strengths beyond their technical skills. "Mission has a strengths-based culture. Our Standout program first identifies each person's unique strengths and then we measure how often that person gets to use his/her strengths every day. We can use this process to match the team member to the right role, and to help team members find meaning in what they do".

Leadership Factors

1. Lack of Physician Leadership

When physician leaders are effective, clinical outcomes are better, while lack of physician leadership is linked to physician burnout and lack of engagement. In 2013, a Mayo Clinic survey of 3,000 physicians found a very strong relationship between physician satisfaction and burnout and the leadership behaviors of physician supervisors in large healthcare organizations (HealthLeaders Media, April 2013).

"I think that what we often do to our clinicians is unfair," said Paulus. "We ask them to have a full clinical load and then expect them to step into leadership roles without any formal training, mentoring, or leadership readiness. That is why we continue to invest in our physician leadership fellowship to support our clinicians so that they can be ready and able leaders. In addition, a few years ago, we started hiring professional medical leaders for our service lines. These leaders are in roles that they want, are qualified for, and make the time to lead and influence."

Having the clinicians in the trenches spending time engaging in small peer-to-peer conversations and dialogue drives satisfaction, engagement, and loyalty among clinicians. That, in turn, reduces burnout and turnover, and eventually extend to other clinical staff beyond physicians, resulting in engagement and a clinical team focused on quality and outcomes. This eventually moves the organization closer to a value-based care.

There are various strategies to use as, again, one size doesn't fit all. So a little later, we'll walk you through a roadmap to engagement. Meanwhile, what are some healthcare organizations doing to drive engagement?

"Engagement is more solid personal communication. When there's good interpersonal communication it facilitates engagement. Engagement comes from people who like to talk because they know how to adjust the conversation to make sure it has a positive impact," Keogh said. Doctors haven't been trained to do that, and they don't necessarily think that talk has much value. Their focus is on the science, the data, hard numbers, and facts.

"Part of the physician problem is that way they are trained," Rosenstein said. "They feel like they're on their own, learning textbook clinical medicine, but learning nothing about how to deal with individuals. Sensitivities are thwarted and brought up in hierarchical situations. But today, you have to be part of a healthcare team and be sensitive to other healthcare workers and to the patients."

The use of science and facts can go far with influencing physicians to become engaged. "Give physicians an opportunity for input," Rosenstein said. "But this is the most important thing.

You must give them an education – the reasons behind a decision to change. You must explain why the change is happening and get them to understand. And the reasons must be based on science or data. They are built on scientific methodology. They are very hard-data oriented. That's what they've been brought up on."

Martin agrees. "You must provide data. Ask them questions such as: 'I've noticed you're taking longer to do these cases, I noticed your infection rate is up, I noticed your patient satisfaction scores are down.' And allow them to respond. You have to present the data and ask them what they think is going on. "And the true test of engagement may be in their reaction: Do they care?"

A survey by Physician Wellness Services and the Cejka Search firm identified the biggest gaps between an ideal engagement situation for physicians and their current status:

- Participation in setting broader organization goals and strategies

- A voice in clinical operations and processes

- Good relationships with administrators

- Fair compensation

- Opportunities for professional development and career advancement

"When we look at the top drivers of engagement, across the board for physicians and employees, they are communication and connection with senior leaders in administration," Rothenberger said. "The difference we see in high-performing organizations is this sense of transparency and inclusion in decision-making."

She added that for both physicians and other healthcare workers, it's not necessarily critical that they be part of setting strategy for the organization. It's more about whether they have the ability to have input on how the strategy is executed.

Keogh believes physicians need to have more teamwork and communication training in their early years of medical school. Since they are still training, medical students may be more willing to "flex" to their non-core strengths.

Rosenstein emphasized the importance of early education, too. He said the process should begin in medical school and residency where, in addition to teaching technical competency skills, physicians should be taught business and personal development skills. If they have those, he said, they will be better prepared for the complexities and challenges they face in their healthcare organizations.

"Seeking collaboration before making a decision may seem tedious and unnecessary to the expert clinician," Keogh stated. "But it is a prerequisite for making organizational decisions, successfully leading teams and getting them to be engaged in their work".

Some medical schools and deans are beginning to recognize the important value of instilling some business, collaboration, and leadership skills in students early on in their medical careers. But others are reluctant to try to cram more material and coursework into curricula that's jam-packed with medical theory and skills development coursework.

Rebekah Apple, PhD, senior manager of programs at the American Medical Student Association, said the type of organization where a medical student lands as a resident plays a role in whether or not physicians are engaged. "Engagement levels may often rely on what residencies folks end up in. A lot of it will depend on where they train and what kind of environment they're training in." She said if it's a top-performing organization where engagement among the physicians and staff is very high, the residents will tend to be more engaged as well.

"They are excited to practice their clinical skills. That is an excitement that can be harnessed," Apple said, but, again, it depends on the organization and how it handles residency training. Apple hasn't necessarily seen many medical schools rushing to incorporate leadership development training in their curricula.

"What medical schools are trying to do more of is infuse a little bit more humanism into the experience and remind medical students why they wanted to become doctors in the first place. And I think maintaining that human element goes a long way toward engagement."

However, some savvy students learn about the importance of engagement on their own. "What I would say is that I am seeing an uptick in students who are creating their own electives in their third year during those rotations where they have the opportunity to do something different," Apple said. "And some of those electives are leadership focused. I definitely think the medical students have a higher level of awareness of the importance of engagement, much more so than their predecessors.

"Having all the information possible at their fingertips [via the Internet], they have knowledge of what the healthcare landscape is going to look like that a physician coming up 20 or 30 years ago did not have coming out of training."

One example of a medical school that is striving to teach personal development, collaboration, engagement, and leadership skills to its medical students is the University of South Florida, Morsani College of Medicine, where I was involved in the formation of the SELECT program for future physician leaders. SELECT stands for Scholarly Excellence Leadership Experiences Collaborative Training.

The SELECT program is best described as follows:

"The program recruits and develops students with the intellectual perspective, empathy, creativity, and passion to change patient care, the health of communities, and the medical profession. The founding principle of SELECT is the concept that students with high emotional intelligence are more likely to develop the skills needed to transform healthcare and improve the health of communities.

In essence: students with a strong foundation in emotional intelligence will become more engaged, compassionate physicians who will connect deeply with their patients and their patients' families; feel more comfortable with and be more effective as team leaders and team members; and have the relationship-building skills and systems perspectives to more effectively lead change in healthcare organizations."

Joann Farrell Quinn, PhD, MBA, who is director of the SELECT competency assessment, said: "the basis of the program is just to make them more effective, more successful and well-rounded physicians." The framework is based on emotional intelligence, and the program lasts through all four years of the students' medical school education. She added that students focus on three different areas:

- Leadership

- Value-based, patient-centered care

- Health systems

For the first three years, students spend about four hours a week in coursework around those topic areas. By the fourth year, it eases back slightly due to the students' busy schedules.

How are students selected for SELECT? USF actually has two distinct programs for medical students, the core program and SELECT. Students must apply for SELECT and go through a screening process to make sure they are a good fit for the program, Quinn explained. "We do behavioral event interviews for the SELECT program. We screen them for signs that they would have a competency in the various emotional/social competencies that we're selecting for."

The SELECT program is in its fifth year. In the first year, just 16 students participated, but the program has grown rapidly and now has about 50 students enrolled each year.

The first two years are spent at USF, then SELECT students spend additional time in their third and fourth years working and studying at the Lehigh Valley Health System in Allentown, Pennsylvania, Quinn said.

Since the program is still relatively young, there's no hard data about its rates of success in producing engaged, teamwork-anchored physicians. Quinn said a longitudinal study recently has been launched to evaluate the program. She emphasized, however, that not all medical students who complete the program will necessarily become physician leaders.

"We're trying to impress upon them that this isn't about a future leadership role; it's about doing what you're supposed to do as a citizen of society as well as a physician. As they move through the program, a lot of them find value in what they're learning." The real test will come when they get their first jobs.

2. Lack of Effective Onboarding

Over the past years, physician turnover has accelerated alarmingly. Surveys show more than 20% of physicians change jobs within the second to third year of practice. Many others seek early retirement citing burnout and reimbursement challenges. Migration from private practices to hospitals has increased precipitously leading to increased competition. Unfortunately, few organizations have formalized on-boarding programs that cement commitment and improve engagement and retention. One organization that has improved engagement through structured onboarding is The Iowa Clinic in Des Moines Iowa. The Iowa Clinic created an extended Physician Onboarding Academy to ensure success and cultural integration through a strategy that ensures alignment, engagement, and retention. Physicians belong to an expert culture. Other healthcare professionals, such as nurses, therapists, administrators, and support staff, usually work in groups, tend to avoid conflict, and are not high risk-takers. Physicians, in contrast, tend to be individualistic risk-takers who prize their autonomy. Outside of patient care, they are more likely to be motivated by self-interest than by group values. TIC recognized that cultural transformation was vital to the successful onboarding, alignment engagement, and retention of its new physicians. The Iowa Clinic's Physician Onboarding Academy immersed new physicians in TIC culture and values: Teamwork, Friendliness, Respect, Excellence, and Ownership. Formal mentorship helped new physicians reduce stress and improve productivity. The "expert" individual-contributor culture of the medical profession fosters individual leadership but fails at building organizational leaders. The Physician Onboarding Academy helped these clinical experts step beyond their comfort zones to become organizational leaders. The Iowa Clinic strategic onboarding programs were linked to increased physician satisfaction and engagement, improved direct reporting job satisfaction and organizational alignment, and improved quality and safety metrics.

Likewise, the physicians and researchers we interviewed said the first evaluation of potential engagement should come up during the hiring process.

"When we interview physicians, we look for a physician who agrees with the institutional mission," Cors, at Lehigh Valley Hospital, said. "We've adopted a much more behavioral-based interview process and offer open-ended scenarios such as asking a candidate to tell us about a difficult communication they've had or about a dispute with a colleague.

"As they talk and give their answers, I'm looking for their integrity, a sense of respect, a sense of teamwork. We don't want to hire lone rangers who never interact with anyone."

Rosenstein also emphasized the importance of onboarding. "Do an onboarding process where you actually talk and meet with a physician and show them you value their work, and they are a vital employee and that you'll help them move through the change." He added that a good example is the need for accurate coding and notes in electronic medical records. Some physicians loathe spending so much time entering data in a computer and say it diminishes the quality of the patient encounter.

But Rosenstein said administrators need to take the time to show physicians how important that data is to reimbursement, while simultaneously empathizing with the physicians and acknowledging the extra burden the EMR sometimes creates.

However, even a strong interviewing and onboarding process doesn't guarantee success. "We had a physician who went through the interview. We thought we had done a good job of screening the physician, and, quite frankly, it was hell from day one," Cors said.

"In a very short period of time, that physician ticked off all the colleagues and we had numerous interventions, explained expectations and mission, vision and values, and we finally ended up saying, 'I'm sorry, you're gone.'" And it wasn't simply a sad situation for the physician, he added. "It's a failure for the physician and a failure for us. It's painful, but it also, in a perverse kind of way, sent a message to others in the organization about the seriousness of engagement."

Personal Factors

Several personal factors that affect engagement: reaching retirement, stress and burnout, lack of time, and energy.

1. Physician Retirement

Instead of dealing with all the hassle factors, finding time and energy to engage in various initiatives *du jour*, physicians are electing to exit the practice. The Association of American Colleges predicts one-third of all physicians will be turning in their white coats and stethoscopes for retirement by 2020. This is a loss of talent, mentorship, and intellect.

SUPPLY VERSUS DEMAND: ALL PHYSICIANS

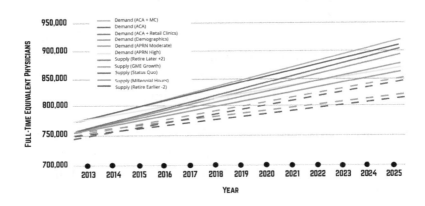

2. Lack of Time and Energy

It is often assumed that physicians are less engaged because they don't have time. They are working in a very hectic environment. Physicians work 14 or 15 hours a day and sometimes remain on call overnight. Every minute at home has become more precious. Being asked to be engaged without having administrative or protective time is difficult to sustain.

Willie Lawrence, MD, knows this all too well.

Lawrence, chief of cardiology at Research Medical Center in Kansas City, Missouri, typically arrives at work around 6 a.m. He makes rounds to see his patients, has meetings at 7 a.m., then spends much of the day seeing new patients, completing catheterizations or other heart procedures, and rounds again on his patients in the 400-bed inner-city hospital.

Fourteen or 15 hours later, he heads home where sometimes he remains on call overnight. "It's tight," he said in a telephone interview that took several calls and emails over four days to schedule. "I don't have administrative days. I don't have time for that. There's no designated time for paperwork. You work it in when you can. Everything happens in between meetings and patient care. You're burning the candle at both ends all the time."

The lifestyle is all-consuming. When he's on-call, he can't be more than 20 to 25 minutes away from the hospital in case an emergency arises such as a heart attack patient who needs immediate care.

Lawrence has spent more than 25 years in practice, first in private practice with a group of cardiologists, and now, as an employed physician of the hospital. He said his passion is caring for patients and sometimes saving a life.

Does he care about quality metrics? Does he follow evidence-based protocols? Does he think about the bigger system-wide problems that the healthcare organization faces? You bet.

But is he what you'd call an engaged physician?

"We are very much engaged and aware of the fact that we are being measured and our outcomes are being made public. We measure everything, including patient satisfaction," he explained. Yet, he knows how some physicians can become disengaged. "The schedule is tough and unpredictable. Some people prefer to have a very structured schedule and they sometimes get disengaged and disenchanted with their employer." Lawrence said he's seen this in some younger millennial physicians who want a lifestyle that's less job-focused. To illustrate how things have changed since he was a young resident, Lawrence said he sometimes attends career events where medical students talk to physicians in various specialties.

In his day, the cardiology table drew lots of traffic, along with those for surgery, trauma care, and other intensive specialties. Today, he said with a chuckle, "the dermatology table is packed and very busy. And I'm sitting there sort of all alone."

Michael Hein, MD, MS, MHCM, a physician leader who's worked in several healthcare organizations and was most recently the CEO of Enhance Health Network in Lincoln, Nebraska, agreed that the busy schedules physicians work these days often don't leave them time to engage in other activities. "My experience has been that the majority of physicians do want to be engaged, but when you put on them the additional administrative burdens that have occurred over the last five or 10 years... that's added several hours of work to a physician's day. And of course, these physicians have families, many of them young families, and so they're liable to say, 'Yeah, I want to be engaged in the quality agenda at the hospital, but I don't have any more time to give."

It's not only time that's lacking, but energy, according to Hein: "There's simply not enough time left in the day for providers to give, and that also includes emotional energy." He added that a sort of "language barrier" adds to the problem of achieving engagement.

The administrative side often uses a different language to describe situations and problems they are trying to tackle. "So we are challenged with breaking that communications gap, too," Hein said.

Jeffrey Moreadith, MD, the chief of acute medicine at Mission Health System in western North Carolina agreed that time is the enemy when it comes to engaging physicians. "It does take a carve-out of time to have the mental space and energy to engage." Luckily, he added, his health system realizes that and gives up-and-coming physician leaders the time to dedicate to administrative efforts such as quality improvement. That extra time can be used to acquire the skills to address administrative issues. "It's much different than solving clinical problems with a patient. Hospitals or system-level problems are more difficult to tackle and must have a different skill set to do that." He added that the physicians themselves need to actually *want* to be involved in the big picture of running a hospital or health system.

"It's time allotment with physicians recognizing that if they don't jump in and participate they're going to be told what to do and there will be no physician input. If I want to be involved, I must carve out time and be compensated appropriately," for taking the steps to engage in administrative-level projects, he said.

Let's now discuss how stress and burnout impact engagement.

How Do Stress and Burnout Impact Engagement?

Nearly 55 percent of physicians are experiencing signs of burnout. Such significant amounts of stress and burnout can lead to cynicism, irritability, apathy, fatigue, dissatisfaction and even severe behavioral disorders or thoughts of suicide (Shanafelt, Hasan, Dyrbye, Sinsky, Satele and others, 2015). More to come later on this issue.

One of the biggest factors that erode engagement is the stress and burnout many physicians experience. The concept of "burnout" is a relatively new one in the annals of human history. Peasants, in medieval times, for example had no such concept. You worked or you were in serious trouble. It was only after two World Wars and the 1960s that human beings began to acknowledge burnout.

The current statistics regarding physician burnout indicate that hospitals and health systems must take action in order to continue to thrive.

- 82 percent of healthcare CEOs surveyed said that physician burnout is growing and only 36 percent said their organization had adopted programs to address burnout (Modern Healthcare, September 2016).

- A 2014 survey of 7,000 physicians by AMA and Mayo Clinic found that nearly 55 percent of physicians were experiencing signs of burnout. Such significant amounts of stress and burnout can lead to cynicism, irritability, apathy, fatigue, dissatisfaction, and even severe behavioral disorders or thoughts of suicide (Shanafelt, Hasan, Dyrbye, Sinsky, Satele and others, 2015).

- In 2013, a Mayo Clinic survey of 3,000 physicians found a very strong relationship between physician satisfaction and burnout and the leadership behaviors of physician supervisors in large healthcare organizations (HealthLeaders Media, April 2103).

Since 2001, the U.S. government's Agency for Healthcare Research and Quality (AHRQ), part of the U.S. Department of Health and Human Services, has been conducting research studies on physician stress and burnout.

One AHRQ-funded project, the MEMO—Minimizing Error, Maximizing Outcome—Study (AHRQ grant HS11955), found that more than half of primary care physicians report feeling stressed because of time pressures and other work conditions. Also contributing to stress and burnout are chaotic environments, low control over work pace, and a poor organizational culture.

The Symptoms

Stress and burnout can lead to cynicism, irritability, apathy, fatigue, dissatisfaction, and even severe behavioral disorders or thoughts of suicide. Just how widespread is the problem of disruptive behavior among physicians?

A 2009 survey of more than 2,100 physicians and nurses about instances of bad behavior found that:

- 30 percent experienced bad or disruptive behavior several times a year.

- Another 30 percent said bad behaviors occurred weekly.

- And 25 percent witnessed disruptive behavior about every month.

Sadly, a whopping 98 percent of the survey respondents reported witnessing behavior problems between doctors and nurses in the past year. (Johnson, 2009.)

Some of the behaviors detailed in the article were beyond the pale:

- Surgical tools and other objects flung across operating rooms.

- Physicians groping nurses and technicians.

- Personal grudges interfering with patient care.

- Accusations of incompetence or negligence expressed in front of patients and their families.

Clearly, in instances like these, engagement has morphed into a verbal and physical engagement of a very different sort.

Immediate action such as suspension, counseling, and intense one-on-one coaching is needed. The engagement is off, and, indeed, the perpetrators and the healthcare organization may be headed for divorce.

Hopefully, these are not routine situations at your healthcare organization. But as you can see, stress, burnout and disengagement can eventually lead to these sorts of bad behaviors, which is yet another reason why healthcare organizations need to focus intently on creating a healthy, engaged workforce.

Combating Burnout

"Burnout is fundamentally an outcome of repetitive frustration," said Ron Paulus, president and CEO of Mission Health in Asheville,

NC. Ron's team has put programs in place to help reduce physician stress and burnout. He added: "It is particularly difficult when there is a disconnect between expectations and reality. The larger the gap, the higher the level of frustration and the greater the probability of progressing to burnout. At Mission, we are approaching wellbeing from a more comprehensive approach." They refer to it as the three-legged stool that includes: 1) System Redesign: "We call it reNEW. How do you take the inefficiency out of the system and out of people's way so they can practice and deliver the best possible and safest care? 2) Having a strength-based culture, and 3) Self-care through LifeXT. "Our Life XT program provides Mission with the necessary tools to increase resilience to stress in order to maximize productivity, focus, and in the end, experience more joy. To reduce burnout, most importantly, again, you need to spend time on matching the expectations to the reality of today's world of healthcare. Many people who are frustrated have large gaps between their expectations and reality."

AHRQ's studies also looked at ways to reduce burnout. We've taken these recommendations, along with our own findings, and organized them into three categories of personal, cultural, and organizational interventions. These suggestions, if adopted and implemented by physicians and organizations, can help alleviate and/or prevent physician burnout.

Personal Interventions

- Pursuing self-awareness and mindfulness training

- Saying no to requests when a person feels overwhelmed

- Establishing healthy boundaries between work and non-work life areas

- Lowering stress by learning effective leadership skills and exerting control wherever possible over one's work hours

- Expressing gratitude each morning when waking up

Cultural/Leadership Interventions

- Stating an organizational intention to value, track, and support physician well-being

- Establishing monthly meetings with providers to talk about work/life issues (frequent communication)

- Connecting with a mentor

- Organizing social events and get-togethers

- Practicing Appreciative Inquiry (identifying what is working well)

- Allowing physicians time to volunteer in the community

- Reconnecting to what matters - developing a strategy

- Sending handwritten thank-you cards

Organizational/System Interventions

Similar to Mission Health's ReNew system approach, assessing, measuring, and reducing hassle factors has proven to reduce stress and improve physician engagement and satisfaction. In a study conducted by CTI, hassle factors in a hospital system and a physician group practice showed that the top three most reported hassles by physicians were:

1. Time spent on Electronic Health Record documentation

2. Demand on the physician time for improving productivity

3. Having collaboration and engagement by peers and colleagues.

Some successful strategies to reduce hassle factors and system related stressors include:

- Employing scribes to take notes for the physicians.

- Creating standing order sets.

- Providing time in the workday and workflow to complete required documentation

- Offering flexible or part-time work schedules

- Hiring floating clinicians to cover gaps

- Instituting regular monitoring for physician burnout amongst providers

- Providing time and funding for physician support meetings

- Supporting flexible work hours

- Providing leadership skills training so they can lead and collaborate with others effectively

- Time and commitment management skills

- Offering confidential coaching for physicians

- Helping physicians develop innovation skills that enable them to rethink and redesign their daily work flow and practice

Grace Terrell, MD, founder and strategist of the 200-physician Cornerstone Health Care in North Carolina, said having physicians as leaders of her practice since it was founded in 1995 is one key to ensuring engagement.

Indeed, if you Google "Cornerstone Health Care High Point, NC" the main link to the group reads: "Cornerstone Health

Care: Physician Led. Patient Driven." And when you click on the board of directors' link, 10 of the 11 directors sport an "MD" after their names.

"The physicians are in complete ownership in our organization. It's not just having them be listened to, it's having them be true leaders in the organization," Terrell explained. The group pays physicians stipends to sit on or lead committees. It empowers them to solve the problems they encounter using innovative ideas and approaches. "You've got to make medicine joyful for physicians again. We allowed them the freedom to come up with ways to provide care that's more focused on patient care than churn in the office."

Rosenstein echoed that idea: "We need to consider physicians as a precious resource and do what we can to understand their concerns and help them rekindle their passion for care."

Indeed, finding joy in the practice of medicine—healing hurts and caring for others in need—is one of the primary reasons students are drawn to medical school. Pranay Sinha, MD, an internal medicine resident wrote in a posting for the popular blog, KevinMD, on September 18, 2017, about how he manages to rekindle joy in his own practice even when things get rough.

"Medical training is no joy ride. How could it be? First, there is the intellectual challenge of cramming knowledge into one's brain and tempering it with good reasoning. Next, there is the physical toll of long hours in the hospital. Most challenging of all is the inescapable spiritual and moral distress in the land of the sick and dying," Sinha wrote (*KevinMD.com-2017*).

Nevertheless, Sinha explains that joy is in the background of practicing medicine every day. "Finding nuggets of happiness in the daily grind of residency need not be complicated. Everyone has a way. Some practice appreciative inquiry by being curious about the people around them and being prompt with their praise: 'That's a cool tattoo. Tell me about it!' or 'Did you see how artfully Dr. Wu explained the plan to the patient?' Others may opt for mindfulness, journaling, or poetry. Really, the method is less important than the desire, nay, determination, to find joy," he wrote.

The American Board of Internal Medicine Foundation website includes videotaped interviews from 2012 about finding joy in the practice of medicine, particularly primary care, which is known for grueling unpredictable hours, flawed models of care, and lower pay than most specialties.

In one of the videos, Christine Sinsky, MD, of Medical Associates Clinic and Health Plans, explores the topic of joy in primary care practices. Among the ideas and innovations that practices are putting into place to ease the burden on primary care providers and rekindle the joy of patient care include:

- Sharing of care with nurses and assistants—emphasizing the team-based model of care

- Cutting down on documentation by hiring scribes (such as www.physicianscribes.org)

- Reengineering the prescription renewal process to move it out of the practice

- Better email management, more verbal messaging, and warm hand-offs improved overall communication among the team and calmed the avalanche of electronic communications

These, along with other practice innovations, relieved pressures on the physicians and the rest of the medical staff, bringing more joy to all those who work in the various clinics where the changes were implemented (*ABIM Foundation videos-2012*).

Those sorts of innovations and changes in practice to restore joy hit home for many doctors who, once again, went into the profession to help patients. At Cornerstone, value-based patient care helps improve working conditions for physicians, as well. The group was one of the early adopters of value-based care. "By 2010, we were using the term 'value' before anyone else knew what it was," Terrell said.

She explained that board meetings and committee meetings always start with a patient story. Sometimes they are good stories and sometimes they aren't. But that simple gesture continually reinforces the group's total focus on patient-centered care. In the end, Terrell said, there are three critical keys to physician engagement: "Focusing the physicians on patient stories and listening to their concerns can make a big difference, and having them be part of the governance structure are the main things that drive engagement."

Terrell also reiterated the idea that allowing physicians to work in areas where they excel and where they have a passion is important to their well-being. Cors shared an example of that as well. He said a rural area of their system's Pennsylvania coverage area had gone for three years without a permanent physician because no one wanted to live in the sparsely populated countryside. Physicians preferred the urban and suburban areas with more attractions and amenities.

Then along came a perfect candidate—a physician who loved the outdoors and immediately fell in love with the idea of living and working in a rural place. "He's now been with us a year," Cors said. "He's out in the woods and we're serving that very rural market that we hadn't served before. If I had put this guy in a big office space in suburbia, he would have freaked out."

So how do we achieve engagement in healthcare organizations, particularly among busy and young physicians? Now that you have a background and understanding of engagement, let's take a look at my step-by-step roadmap to improve physician engagement.

Engagement Roadmap

Now, open Google Maps and search for "physician engagement roadmap."

Here's the message that came up when I looked it up:

"We could not find *physician engagement roadmap*. Make sure your search is spelled correctly. Try adding a city, state, or zip code."

Nope.

Up until now, there's been no clear roadmap to physician engagement.

Sure, there are various strategies to consider when attempting to improve physician engagement: take more surveys, ask managers to come up with a plan, hire a consultant, offer additional perks, beg and cheerlead in the hallways and physician lounges. But what truly works? And what doesn't?

As with any important initiative, getting from the current state to the desired state requires a clear strategy – a roadmap. Having worked with hundreds of healthcare leaders and thousands of physicians, this is what I have found to work.

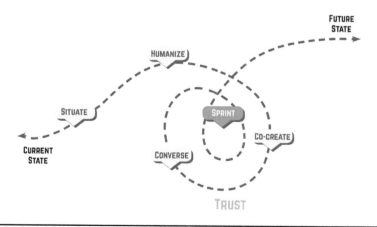

This roadmap to physician engagement is a powerful tool that will help you achieve higher engagement through a step-by-step process that is simple, counterintuitive, and results in positive, measurable outcomes.

Context First

As we discussed earlier in this book, engagement is not one size fits all. Engagement should not be an initiative. It should be an enabler of all initiatives. Engagement should not be a metric to chase. Engagement should be part of the culture—how we get things done in healthcare. Engagement is contextual, is a leadership act, a linguistic act, and is a choice. Engagement has to be an intentional effort.

First, you need to be selective and focus your efforts. You need to identify where you need engagement the most to succeed. What are the strategic priorities that depend on active and effective physician engagement? Common priorities we hear from healthcare leaders include:

- Implementing evidence-based practices (three-hour sepsis bundle)

- Participation in committees such as peer review, MEC, department, quality

- Improving quality, safety agenda

- Improving patient experience

- Implementing interdisciplinary rounding

- Reducing variations in practices and outcomes

- Reducing cost of care

- Improving hand-off between providers

Let's take the first step of the Journey with Situate......

Step 1: Situate

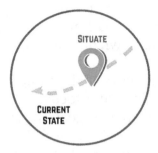

Effective leaders and strategists must know their terrain first... Different terrains require different strategies...

-Sun Tzu, The Art of War

Imagine planning to take a cross-country road trip. Engagement, like such a trip, is a journey. It's not a quick drive across town to a shopping center. It's a long ride with several stops along the way. How would you prepare for a cross-country road trip? You'd most likely prepare by mapping the terrain.

What types of traffic will you encounter? City stop-and-go traffic, or high-speed interstate driving? What does the weather look like? Will you run into storms or snow? Or will you be driving through the desert under grueling heat? Is your vehicle fit for the trip? Oil changed? Sturdy tires? Windshield wiper fluid?

Just like preparing for the trip, the first stop on the roadmap to physician engagement begins by situating and assessing the terrain, defining the future and desired situation and where your physicians stand when it comes to engagement today versus where you need them to be.

Different terrains require different strategies. To take just one survey of all physicians/clinicians in an organization every other year and try to come up with an engagement strategy to engage all physicians is a tall order. You likely won't succeed, and will suffer a breakdown on the highway, so to speak.

We believe you need to look at engagement as a strategy that's more personalized and focused on a specific strategic, operational or clinical area, or goal. For example, at Lee Health, in Ft. Myers, Florida, Chief Medical Officer and Chief Operating Officer, Scott Nygaard, MD, MBA, assessed that there is direct correlation between physician engagement and systems results. "So goes the physicians, so goes the system," Nygaard said, noting that physicians still hold the reins in healthcare organizations and can heavily influence the culture. "If physicians don't lead to the highest level, then people (the entire staff) are not going to get above that level of performance."

Nygaard decided to focus his engagement strategy on his physicians in the Lee Physician Group. That was his terrain.

There is tremendous value in focusing your strategy. Sun Tzu in the Art of War said: *Focus targets a specific way to advance your position by filtering the unnecessary activities.*

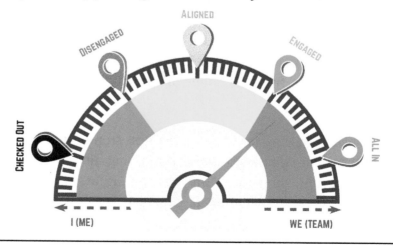

When the approach is focused, your chances of success are higher since you are dealing with a finite, manageable terrain.

You can assess the terrain more effectively to gauge where everybody stands.

1. Whose engagement do you need in order for the initiative to succeed?

2. Who could block or derail the change if not "engaged?"

3. Who will be impacted and/or involved in implementation?

Next, for each physician or physician groups, assess:

1. Their current level of engagement – all-in and energized versus actively disengaged.

2. Desired level of engagement – where do you need them to be?

3. How critical they are to the success of your initiative?

Situating yourself in the terrain, you can identify which physicians are all in. You're looking for true partners and innovators. I like to call them "mo-joes." Here are the kinds of behaviors you see from them:

- Optimism

- Can-do attitude

- A sense of altruism

- Ownership

- Pleasant to be around

- Ready to act

- Frustrated by lack of actions

Which physicians fall into the neutral silent majority? These physicians are neither highly engaged nor disengaged. They go at their daily work and don't care.

Which physicians are actively disengaged or even resisters? I call them "no-joes," and they are the disengaged physicians who are likely to be your greatest challenge if you let them. They usually are:

- Dramatic

- Loud

- Playing the victim

- Complaining

- Blame

- Walking in place

- Cynical

- Pessimistic

- Painful to be around

- Passive aggressive

- Not showing up to meetings/lack commitment

Typically, the normalized distribution of engaged, silent, and disengaged physicians breakdown is as follows:

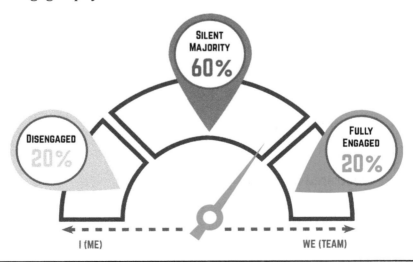

- 20 percent of physicians are typically actively engaged and all in (mo-joes)

- 20 percent are disengaged or resisters (no-joes)

- And the majority, 60 percent, are silent (don't care and going about their day)

The common mistake made by leaders is that they spend 80 percent of their time focusing on the 20 percent who are disengaged because leaders often feel they need to fix everything and/or because, typically, these physicians are the loudest. While there are situations where you have to focus on the disengaged (when they are very connected influencers who are very critical to the success of the initiative/organization), try to look at the situation differently.

While the leader is reacting and focusing his or her energy and time on the disengaged or the loudest, the fence sitters, who are the silent majority, are getting mixed leadership signals and would elect to wait to act or commit. Even worse, the already engaged and committed physician may get frustrated or disappointed due to the lack of attention and distraction of the leader.

It may seem a bit counterintuitive, but leaders who focus their energy and time on those who are already engaged and all-in get better leverage and success than other leaders. When you work with those who are already engaged and you support them, you solidify your positive opportunities in the terrain, and these physicians will eventually influence their peers in the silent majority, including some of the disengaged.

To give you a better understanding of how mapping the terrain would work in a real-life scenario, let's look at a team of hospitalists at one of the largest health system in the country – Catholic Health Initiative (CHI). Catholic Health Initiatives

(CHI) is a non-profit, faith-based health system established in 1996. It operates in 18 states with 96 hospitals, 4 academic health centers and teaching hospitals, and 26 critical-access facilities, community health-services organizations, accredited nursing colleges, and home health agencies.

CHI leaders decided to make sepsis the focus of a hospital-wide patient safety campaign to improve compliance with the bundles and simultaneously improve the organization's hospital quality scores and outcomes. A group of hospitalists were given the task to improve physician engagement in sepsis bundle compliance in order to save lives.

Sepsis accounts for one-third to one-half of deaths that occur in U.S. hospitals each year—an estimated 225,000 to 350,000 deaths. Some patients arrive at hospitals already suffering from sepsis. Others contract it during their stay. It can affect all age groups and is particularly deadly for those who have compromised immune systems and are more susceptible to infection. Sepsis can strike quickly and without much warning, and it can escalate fast, resulting in a major infection overnight.

Hospitals are having success combating sepsis by following certain protocols—or sepsis bundles—whenever the infection is suspected. Typically, a sepsis bundle includes:

- Taking a blood sample to measure lactate, a byproduct of turning blood sugar into energy; high serum lactate level is a sign of severe metabolic distress

- Culturing the blood to identify infection

- Starting the patient on a broad-spectrum antibiotic

- Keeping the patient well hydrated

Here's the rub. Although the bundle has been proven to work, some physicians still won't follow the protocol.

Some may refuse to believe that their patient has sepsis, especially if they are in the hospital for a routine procedure. Others don't catch the warning signs early enough. Some may not believe the bundles are an effective way to treat sepsis.

Yes, it's a problem of engagement – a problem that our roadmap can help alleviate.

The team at CHI adapted the engagement roadmap and started their efforts by situating and mapping the terrain at one specific hospital. They identified the physicians who were highly engaged, cared about safety, and employed sepsis bundles routinely and labeled them green. They also identified the physicians and/or leaders that were also critical to the success of the sepsis initiative. Then, they identified those in the silent majority who may or may not be complying with the protocols and/or supporting the efforts and labeled them yellow. Finally, they identified those physicians who were disengaged and most likely to reject the sepsis bundles, and determined whether their support was critical and labeled them red. Next, and most critically, the team had to have an honest and courageous conversation (call it healthy debate) to assess how critical each physician or group was for the success of the sepsis initiative. The more critical they were, the more attention and focus they had to put on that physician or group of physicians.

Next the hospitalists needed to identify where they needed the engagement level to be at for each physician or group so that they could be successful in their endeavors.

Their map of the terrain looked like this:

SEPSIS ENGAGEMENT MAP

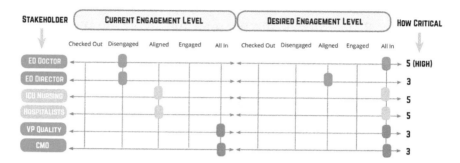

The result of the SITUATE activities was clarity, focus, and better utilization of the team's time and resources.

Summary of Actions - SITUATE

☐ Define your terrain

o Don't spread yourself too broad and too thin. Engagement is contextual.

☐ Assess your terrain

o Identify all the key stakeholders and physicians that are critical to your initiative success.

o For each of the stakeholders and physicians, map where their engagement level related to your initiative or goal (Green, yellow, and red).

o For each of the stakeholders and physicians, map where you need their engagement level to be at for your initiative to be successful.

☐ Identify who is critical to your success.

o Assess how critical each stakeholder or physician is to your initiative success

☐ Focus your energy and resources on the critical physicians or staff.

o Select who is critical and requires your focus, energy, time, and attention.

Step 2: Humanize

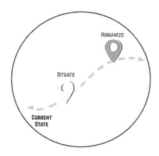

Randy Haffner Ph.D. President/CEO of the Multi-State Division for AdventHealth has dedicated his professional life to faith-based healthcare, leading organizations like the Florida Hospital in Orlando, Florida, and Porter Adventist Hospital in Denver, Colorado. Randy has a great gift of connecting with his physicians by humanizing the conversation. What is more human than a father telling him and his wife Cindy's personal story of the challenging birth of their first daughter Bailey? I watched Randy tells the story to a room full of physicians and bringing some of them to tears in the process.

Randy's wife, Cindy, went into pre-term labor three months early at only 27 weeks of gestation. After scanning with ultrasound, and Cindy being stabilized, the perinatologist discovered that the baby had duodenal astria, where the first part of the small intestine is totally blocked limiting the digestion of amniotic fluid and causing pre-term labor. Cindy was confined to bed rest for ten weeks.

Randy continues: *"At 37 weeks, Cindy went into labor. During birth, the fetal monitoring equipment began sending warning signals. The concern was obvious in the obstetrician's face. With the baby stuck in the birth canal, it was too late for delivery by caesarian section. After many attempts, our daughter made her first appearance into the world. Cindy and I waited breathlessly for the baby's first cry. Our hearts pounded in our chests as we looked for some sign of the baby's pulse. But she was ashen and limp. We'd already given her a name, Bailey. But Cindy couldn't hold our firstborn in her arms. The staff whisked our daughter away immediately to the neonatal team. They began their work with great clinical precision and expertise."*

Every newborn is evaluated on an Apgar Scale that quantifies an infant's overall health on a scale of one to ten. Heart rate, skin complexion, respiration, reflexes and muscle tone are all assessed. Normal healthy babies score in a range of seven to ten. Bailey scored a one.

Randy Continued: *"I still vividly remember sitting with the neonatologist, Dr. Eduardo Lugo, as he explained the severity of the situation. He described in detail that our daughter had very little blood volume in her body. Although not diagnosed, the likelihood was a bleed in the brain. It was heartbreaking news. And yet, I could still sense the caring and the empathy in his voice. Dr. Lugo had to tell us that it was unlikely Bailey would make it through the night. And even if she did, she had little chance of becoming a normal, healthy child. And yet he didn't deliver this as simply scientific information. **There was a real human being there, talking to another human being who was dangling on the edge of fatherhood.** As the physicians and nurses swarmed around our daughter, providing state-of-the-art critical care medicine, a separate group of caregivers and chaplains focused their love and attention on Cindy and me. They spoke with us at the appropriate times. They prayed with us. They helped us get in touch with the love and strength that only God can provide in situations like these. They helped create an atmosphere of trust. Through it all, they created something I can only call the **"spirit of medicine."***

At the end, it all turned out ok. Today, Bailey has grown to be a healthy, successful young lady about to get married at the time of the publishing of this book.

Similar to Randy's story, we have to humanize the conversation about the clinical or business issue we like others to engage in. We have to connect the conversation to a noble cause or purpose that others would relate to and connect with, like saving lives. For example, instead of talking about sepsis bundle compliance, we talk about saving a loved one's life. We make it human. We connect with the head and the heart of the other person or physician. When we humanize the conversation, our body releases oxytocin, which helps improve trust.

Let's look at the following relationships:

To get results from others, we need actions. To get meaningful actions, we need a change in behaviors. To change behaviors, we need a change in mindsets; to change mindsets, we need to understand their underlying assumptions. Mindsets are below the water in an iceberg.

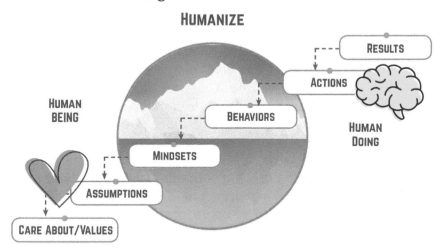

Typically, we see actions and behaviors of others – the human doing side. We often see or hear the following:

- I don't need to change
- I don't trust the data

- I don't have time

- This is not relevant to me

- My patients are different, sicker, and more complex

Other signs of disengagement are:

- Exhibiting distrust of others or the organizations

- Not showing up for critical meetings

- Not responding to communication

- Disruptive behavior

To really engage physicians, you need to humanize the conversation and align the desired outcome to what the clinicians really care about and connect to their personal values. That requires you to see each person as a human being versus a human doing, and to get a deeper understanding and connection with every individual you have identified as critical to achieving the desired outcome.

Seeing the physician as a human being first allows you to be more open and curious about what he or she cares about and his or her sources of disengagement. When you do that, you get to see that there are many likely sources of disengagement, including purpose, individual level, cultural level, leadership, and system level.

For example, on the purpose level, physicians will pay attention to what they care about, such as patient care. Meaning and value occur when there is an intersection between your request, actions, what they are concerned about, what they care about, and what their values are.

VALUE DOES NOT START UNTIL THERE IS A BREAKDOWN

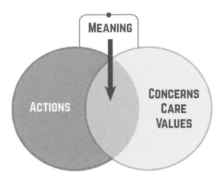

On an individual level, it could be the lack of mastery skills to perform the duties conducive to achieving the goals; or, it could be the lack of will, or simply not wanting to engage or change behaviors. After all, engagement is a choice. In this case, you have to decide if that is okay. In his book, *Drive: The Surprising Truth About What Motivates Us*, Daniel Pink documented that professionals are motivated intrinsically in three different ways: autonomy, mastery, and purpose (Pink-2012,). It is not enough to talk about burning platforms; we need to connect with people's burning ambitions, motivations, purposes and desires.

On the cultural level, it could be the surrounding social network where "no-joes" are the loudest and are enforcing rules that won't allow the changes and improvements to take place. Another source of disengagement could be the incentives you have that reward the wrong behaviors. For example, we like our physicians to focus on patient experience, and yet, a typical reward system based on RVU (Relative Value Unit) rewards volume versus experience. On the leadership level, the source of disengagement could be the lack of effective clinical leadership that listens to the physician concerns. On the system level, the source of disengagement could be the increase in hassle factors and the increased complexity of the structures and processes in place.

DISENGAGEMENT FACTORS

Assess the root cause of disengagement

PURPOSE	SELF/PERSON	CULTURAL	LEADERSHIP	SYSTEM
• Lack of ownership • Lack of alignment • Lack of autonomy • Lack of meaning	• Lack of skill or lack of will • Lack of energy or time • Stress and burnout	• Lack of trust • Conflicting cultures • Generational differences	• Lack of effective clinical leadership and support • Dysfunctional medical staff • Lack of understanding	• Hassle factors in the way • Complexity of structure and/or problems that get in the way

This is what Damian (Pat) Alagia III, MD, MBA, found out when he tried to understand the factors impacting his physician's engagement. Pat served as Chief Physician Executive and Chief Medical Officer from 2013 to 2016 at KentuckyOne Health, a $2.5 billion health system, in Kentucky.

When he arrived, he conducted a physician engagement survey that placed KentuckyOne in the 10th percentile. "It was very low, not a good situation," Alagia said. In other words, the map of the terrain was tattered and torn.

After studying the situation and talking to physicians, Alagia identified seven factors that correlated with physician dissatisfaction and disengagement:

Leadership Factors	1. The administrators and executives' ability to manage and engage physicians in the strategic direction of the hospital
	2. Responsiveness to physician concerns
Cultural Factors	3. Communication with physicians
	4. Physician involvement with decision making
System Factors	5. The safe care of patients
	6. Consistency in the delivery of healthcare services
	7. Inclusion in quality improvement

Based on these findings, he explained, the overarching message was one of transparency, accountability, inclusion, and collaboration.

It is at this point on the engagement roadmap that you must take the time to assess and understand those physicians' mindsets and assumptions. You need to figure out what narrative is running through the physicians' minds about you or the proposed initiative or change, and then find ways to allay those assumptions or fears. Remember, they are scientists who start with skepticism and would prefer facts and evidence over subjective conjecture.

IDENTIFY ASSUMPTIONS

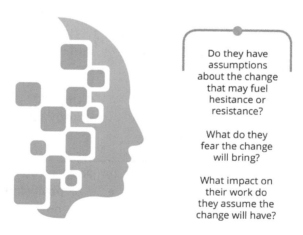

Do they have assumptions about the change that may fuel hesitance or resistance?

What do they fear the change will bring?

What impact on their work do they assume the change will have?

You are probably telling yourself, *I don't have time for all of this discovery*. That is exactly my point: if you don't invest the time on an ongoing basis to know and connect with your physicians as human beings, you will not achieve engagement.

By taking the time to know physicians' assumptions and motivators, you can powerfully humanize and align the conversation to a common purpose.

IDENTIFY KEY MOTIVATIONS
Why *They* Would Care About the Change

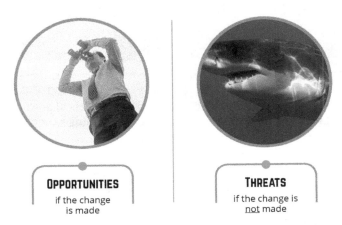

OPPORTUNITIES	THREATS
if the change is made	if the change is not made

Let's look at our sepsis example. What opportunities, especially those that directly affect physicians, will be gained by following the sepsis bundles?

- Patients will get better sooner and experience a shorter length of stay

- Patients won't die from the infections

- There's a lower risk to the practice

- The physician's ego and reputation won't be damaged by experiencing a patient death

- The physician's patient satisfaction scores are better protected

- The hospital's morbidity ratings are not impacted

- There's a potential for better reimbursement in shared risk/shared saving

- The hospital's reputation won't suffer a blow, so it will stay competitive

SEPSIS - HUMANIZE

THREATS (if not applied)	OPPORTUNITIES (if applied)
• Longer length of stay • Higher risk of practice • **LIVES ARE IMPACTED** • Reimbursement in shared risk/shared saving • Diminished ability to compete • Reputation	• Shorter length of stay • Lower risk of practice • **LIVES ARE SAVED** • Better reimbursement in shared risk/shared saving • Better ability to compete • Better patient management and referrals.

And the threats if sepsis bundles are not initiated?

- Longer hospital stays

- High risk to the practice

- More patient deaths

- Lower reimbursement

- Physician and hospital reputations damaged

- Ability to compete diminished

When the hospitalist team changed the conversation from compliance with the three-hour bundle to "saving lives," they were able to connect with what a disengaged physician cares about. Then, he or she began to engage in the conversation, watching more closely for signs of sepsis and using sepsis bundles when infection was suspected.

Summary of Actions - HUMANIZE

☐ Think about the human being before human doing

☐ Understand sources of disengagement

- o Purpose

- o Self/Purpose

- o Cultural

- o Leadership

- o System

☐ Identify what the physicians care about

- o Value occurs when there is an intersection between your actions and what they care about

☐ Identify what are the physicians' assumptions

☐ Identify the physicians' motivators

- o Threats

- o Opportunities

☐ Align your conversation and narrative to what people care about

- o Start with the why, like saving lives

- o Make it personal and human, like Randy did

Step 3: Co-Create

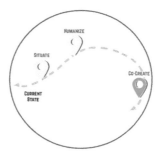

Your next stop on the journey to engagement is crucial to achieving success. *It is critical to move to partnering by realizing that engagement is not a one-way street. It is not just your responsibility to engage the physicians, as they are professionals. As such, they make choices about engaging or not engaging. Co-creation is a form of partnership that builds trust.*

Co-creation is collaborative process to design, generate value, or develop solutions to existing problem. Co-creation is a partnership between equals. This concept is becoming more popular among innovative companies as they co-create with their customers, which leads to better designed products and services. I believe it is essential to use the same concept of partnership to engage the physicians in the healthcare transformation movement.

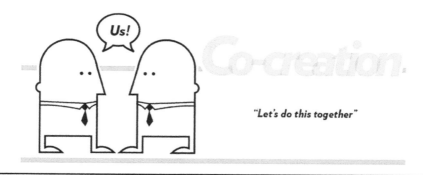

So how do you start a movement? There is a famous and funny TEDx video that shows a guy, at a park, who gets up and starts dancing in full view of others. But nothing happens, and the rest of the crowd ignores him. It is not until a second person joins the public dancing that spectators start noticing. Then, a third person joins and as more and more people join, others that were sitting and watching start to get up and run to join because they don't want to be left out. This all leads to a public dancing movement. The tipping point was the second person's willingness to follow and co-create with the first dancer/leader.

Similarly, the best way to start a movement and momentum of engagement is to form a coalition with the already engaged physicians who are willing to co-create with you and engage their peers to move a process forward.

> Don't think for a minute that you can do it on your own, or through the sheer authority of your position. It's critical that you move from an "I" to "we" mentality and realize that the best way to engage physicians is to not make it "my plan," but "our plan." It's not "my ideas," but "our ideas," and one of the best ways to better engage physicians and others is to ask for help. That's right: the simple act of asking for help is almost guaranteed to bring cooperation from the person you're seeking as a supporter.

By co-creating and asking for help, you're intimating that you need and value their assistance. It's a much more effective way of cooperation compared to telling them they need to get onboard.

So how do you go about building a coalition?

First, and this may sound counter intuitive, you need to engage the natural leaders and the already-engaged physicians and enable them to co-create with you to achieve your goals or complete your projects.

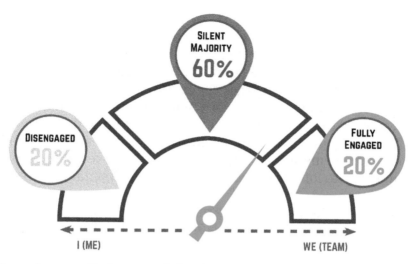

How do you find natural leaders to co-create with you and engage others? Look for physicians on your staff who:

- Are early adopters
- Are interested in what's best for the patients and the collective good
- Are positive and trigger the best instincts in others
- Make the right things matter most
- Create strong authentic connections built on trust
- Seek out and listen to others' input
- Influence and motivate others even when they are not their superiors
- Have high emotional intelligence
- Are open to new ideas
- Exhibit integrity and trust
- Are skillful communicators
- Lift the mood of others

So how do you find the natural leaders? Have you heard of the red car concept? When you decide you want to buy a red car, all of the sudden you start seeing red cars on the road and in parking lots, even though they were there the whole time. When you point your mental compass toward natural leaders and the highly engaged (mo-joes), they will show up for you.

However, identifying natural leaders is not enough. Empowering those natural leaders with the necessary tools is critical to success. You need to help them develop their engagement muscle.

Engagement is a muscle that you have to develop. It's like working out at the gym. It takes repeated efforts over a period of time. Just as there are no magic pills to instantly lose weight or gain muscle strength, there are no quick fixes for achieving engagement. You have to invest in developing natural leaders with a very structured leadership process that gives them the opportunity to co-create so that they can eventually reach out, engage, and influence others.

In my work at CTI, I have found that the best way to develop natural leaders is to give them a structured and well-organized cohort experience. They need to feel the power of a group, and build trust and emotional safety with each other. In addition, they need support through coaching and team projects where they are solving an issue together and exercising those co-creation and engagement muscles with others. Through these exercises, they will build the key skills of "leading self" first, actively listening, leading others through change, having courageous and difficult conversations, and finally, influencing others. It is essential to offer them support, coaching, training, and development opportunities to empower them in dealing with push back and resistance from other physicians. It is important to empower them by giving them the data and the stories and materials needed to make the argument to others.

In fact, in his famous Harvard Business Review article, "Accelerate," HBR November 2012 issue, John Kotter, the Konosuke Matsushita Professor of Leadership, Emeritus at Harvard Business School and the author of 17 books, including

"Leading Change," discusses the importance of having more leadership, not just more management to accelerate change. "At the core of a successful hierarchy is competent management. A strategy network, by contrast, needs lots of leadership, which means it operates with different processes and language and expectations. The game is all about vision, opportunity, agility, inspired action, and celebration—not project management, budget reviews, reporting relationships, compensation, and accountability to a plan." In addition, an army of volunteers should be organized in "two structures, one organization." Establishing a separate structure of an army of volunteers to improve and implement strategies that is not inhibited by the existing traditional hierarchies is a more effective way to accelerate change.

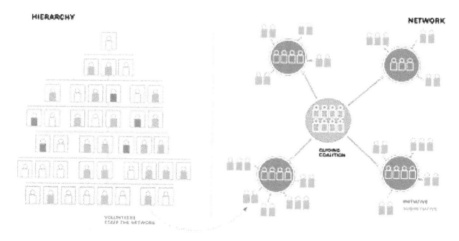

That was the successful strategy used by Dr. Joe Cozzolino, MD, MBA, to build and empower a coalition at Florida Medical Clinic, a 200-physician group practice based in Tampa, Florida. Joe is the Chairman of the Medical Executive Committee at Florida Medical Clinic.

The group's Medical Executive Committee was formed about two years ago to lead the transition from volume to value-based healthcare. It was our way to engage the physicians to co create and solve strategic initiative. However, it was quickly realized that the members lacked the necessary leadership training. "Interestingly, I became the chairman of a group of eight physicians, and the group had no formal leadership training," Cozzolino said.

The committee engaged CTI to help with leadership training and teach the members how to better engage with the other physicians in the practice. "We wanted them to become liaisons to the physicians throughout the group and encourage more engagement," Cozzolino said. He added that the training has been invaluable to jump starting the effort: "We've been at it for a year now, and we're finally beginning to see the fruits of that labor."

Prior to the formation of the executive committee, the board of directors handed down all the decisions about the way the business would be run, Cozzolino explained. But with CTI's guidance, "what we learned through the leadership training is that people accept the change that they help co-create, which was really a revolutionary idea for the clinic." These are examples of steps 1, 2 and 3 on the roadmap: situate, humanize, and co-create.

Specifically, the engagement effort is meant to find consensus about the physicians, end conflict, and embolden the front-line physicians to play a leading role in helping to transform the clinic from volume to value. For example, a cardiologist, who was one of the liaisons, is taking a congestive heart failure disease management program clinic-wide. The pulmonary liaison is doing the same with a chronic obstructive pulmonary disease program. A hypertension management program is being created, too. The group is also rolling out an employee health program for the clinic.

All of these involve physicians who were going through the leadership and physician engagement training, Cozzolino said. "The best part about the training, is being a real-world training that, a year later, delivers real and tangible results."

In addition to developing programs and protocols, the leadership training "has brought a lot of comradery among us, deepened our trust in each other, and it brought us all together … We're going to keep meeting monthly and continue to come up with real-world results over the next year," Cozzolino shared.

"One of the pearls of wisdom that I've learned and seen throughout this training is that you have to show others what is possible," he said, and that as the efforts spread throughout the clinic, other physicians will want to be involved in the change and help create it. "The best part of the training is that you get to take industry-leading ideas and cutting-edge theories and they (CTI) help put it all together for you."

"I think that what we often do to our clinicians is unfair. We ask them to have a full clinical load and then expect them to step into leadership roles without any formal training, mentoring, or leadership readiness," said Dr. Ron Paulus, CEO of Mission Health. Paulus thinks it's not right to throw physicians into leadership roles without any training. "That is why we continue to invest in our physician leadership fellowship to support our clinicians so that they can be ready and able leaders".

At Lee Health, in Ft. Myers, Florida, the CMO, Dr. Scott Nygaard, has been engaging about 25 physicians and non-physician practice leaders through the leadership development program each year for the past five years. Physicians have to apply to participate in the program and every year, there are more applications than spots available, Nygaard said. "We don't have to do any marketing. The physicians themselves are the ones who are selling it to other physicians, telling them about the value of the program."

In this program, which extends over ten months, the group meets monthly to participate in the coaching and coursework and share insights on how their leadership journeys are progressing. They are better prepared to engage effectively in the co-creation of solutions.

He said one key learning point for the participants is strengthening the care teams at the six hospitals that make up Lee Health. "The idea is that we will make better decisions together than we would independently, and we try to stress that in the cohorts that we have here."

Among the projects the cohorts have tackled throughout the years are:

- A better onboarding process for physicians coming onto the staff

- Improved credentialing process

- Stronger communication pathways and creating a shared vision

- How to put performance measures in place

"It's all resulted in better interaction, better engagement, better planning ... and they are engaged and listening better. They're not just showing up to do a job," Nygaard said.

Furthermore, the physicians who complete the leadership training program "walk out of there with a new appreciation for leadership and how to manage and lead a program and how to engage and effectively work together."

Even after the formal leadership training ends, Lee Health periodically brings the cohorts back together to let them refresh their knowledge and share insights. "The idea is to encourage them to continue to build their networks of relationships within the system." Nygaard added that the physicians don't just learn leadership skills exclusive to their jobs. "They walk out of there, out of the training, knowing how to be a better spouse, a better parent, a better citizen, because a lot of what they are learning is what I consider to be life skills."

In the sepsis example, the CHI hospitalist team looked across their organizations to first find the staff and physicians who are supportive and using the sepsis bundle and are actively engaged in applying the protocols. They were the physicians or staff who have been advocating for better management of sepsis. In the chart below, they are the one in green.

SEPSIS ENGAGEMENT MAP

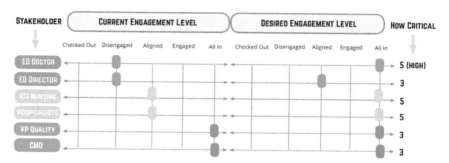

Once they found the supporters and natural leaders, the real work began. They talked to the physicians individually, taking them to breakfast or rounding with them. They took time to build relationships with them by taking interest in them individually as human beings first, and not as "human doings."

The hospitalist team had to ask the coalition what it would take to encourage their peers to care about the bundle. What are the obstacles to get buy-in from others? What can they do to help convince others to use the bundles? Who else can they recommend to be part of the coalition? How do we communicate the opportunities that come with more evidence-based care and/or the threats that result from the lack of bundle adoption? These questions and dialogues led to finding out the need for additional resources to humanize the message to others. These resources included training and peer reviewed articles on the evidence of improved safety and quality when bundles are applied. They also included assembling stories and videos of real families talking about the impact of losing loved ones due to sepsis and/or the stories of saving someone's life due to effective diagnosis and treatment of sepsis.

Summary of Actions – CO-CREATE

☐ Co-Create is about building trust

☐ Be counter intuitive. Engage the already engaged physicians

   o Organize them in a cohort

   o Teach them the necessary skills to lead self and engage others

   o Engage them in meaningful projects

☐ Be intentional about developing your coalition

   o Give them the necessary tools and data

☐ Organize your army of volunteers in "two structures, one organization"

Trust is at the Heart of it

"Trust is the new currency in our interdependent, collaborative world"

Stephen M.R. Covey

As Judith E. Glaser noted in "Conversational Intelligence: How Great Leaders Build Trust and Get Extraordinary Results" "When trust is absent, we see REALITY with threatened eyes, and we reveal less than what we know or what is helpful to move forward, assume the worst of others, become cautious, fearful, and even avoid confronting the truth. *"When we are in a state of distrust, the world feels threatening. Threats make us retreat. They make us feel we need to protect ourselves."*

Think of trust as a bank account we have with our physicians. It includes deposits and withdrawals.

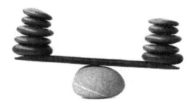

Deposits happen when we as leaders:

1. Are authentic and open

2. Are empathetic with others

3. Include others in decision making

4. Give them autonomy

5. Ask them for input

6. Ask them questions

7. Make them offers of help

8. Express appreciation

9. Share resources and knowledge

10. Recognize them

11. Provide them coaching to help them take their game to the next level.

12. Describe the ideal state that connects with their values and what they care about

13. Engage physicians to create strategies together

14. Be sensitive with the realities and challenges that physicians face

15. Listen

16. Communicate openly and frequently

17. Invest in robust physician leadership development

18. Never abuse your power and authority

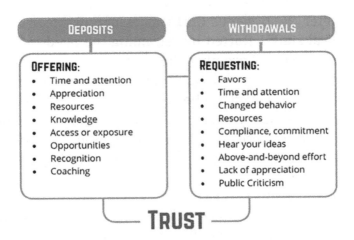

On the opposite end, withdrawals occur when we as leaders:

1. Order someone to do things without explanation or context

2. Order others to change behavior without context

3. Ask others for compliance

4. Don't show appreciation

5. Don't treat physicians as human being first

6. Criticize in public versus private

7. Do something that breaks trust with someone

8. Don't explain the "why" for the shift or change

9. Don't connect the vision to shared values

Trust isn't something that happens quickly. Ron Paulus, MD, CEO, at Mission Health knows this first hand. In fact, Paulus has been working on it for nearly a decade. "I see engagement as a journey and as a multi-level strategy," he explained. "I started this particular journey in 2010 when I arrived to Mission Health, after the previous CEO was essentially thrown out by the medical staff. I started by reframing the need to focus on a common vision: becoming the best in clinical quality and safety in the nation and determining how we could deliver on that vision by ensuring the best outcomes for every patient in our care. Since then, we have been working together with our providers and delivering on this common vision." To build trust and engagement, we established strong guiding principles, which include:

- Patients First: "Above all, through the eyes of our patients and their families, we do what is best."

- Interdependence: "We serve one another and our community best by working collaboratively as partners."

- Benefit of the Doubt: "We willingly offer one another the benefit of the doubt when circumstances are unknown, assuming the best, and yet practice and insist upon Just Culture."

These guiding principles provide common language and ethos with providers and staff at Mission.

When there is trust, we get to see the world with different lenses. As Judith Glazer said, "Trust is the glue that holds an organization together in the face of enormous challenges. Trust primes the pump so that people can get intimate and feel open enough to be inclusive, interactive, and intentional. With Trust, we see reality more clearly and are more open to engage. When we are in a state of trust, we experience reality with new eyes and we reveal more, assume the best of others, look at situations with an open heart, and interpret communications through truth and facts."

At the beginning of the book, we used the formula Strategy X Engagement = Transformative Results. We now can modify this formula to include another multiplier of Trust! Strategy x Engagement X Trust = Transformative Results

Taking stock in how healthy our trust accounts are with physicians is THE critical step of engagement.

Step 4: Converse

George Bernard Shaw once said: "The greatest problem with communication is the illusion that it's being accomplished."

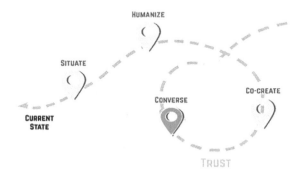

Now you're ready to begin the fourth step on the road to engagement: having the conversation. At this stage you are relying on the coalition of "already engaged natural leaders" to engage and influence the silent majority and even the late adopters. Influence and engagement are linguistic acts. It is through conversations that we establish trust, relationships, influence, and, eventually, engagement.

Already Existing Listening

WHAT DO THEY HEAR?

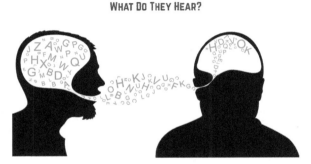

The challenge with communication is that we assume the physician is receiving exactly what we are saying without any filtering, assumption, or interpretation. Unfortunately, that is not the case. Our words, gestures, tones, and body language are all being "heard" through the lens of "Already Existing Listening." Such a filter includes history with us or the organization, trust level, assumptions about the speaker, the issue of discussion, or the organization. It may include interpretations that lead to fears, concerns for self, or feeling threatened.

Asking Versus Telling

When asking for help, the questions you ask are important. By posing the question in a way that solicits their opinions and insights, you better your chances of getting them to engage and give you the help you need.

Indeed, research shows questions are powerful tools for influence. A 2017 article in *Fast Company* titled "Want to Know What Your Brain Does When It Hears a Question?" explores the behaviors behind questions and answers (*Hoffeld-2017*). "Questions are powerful. Not only does hearing a question affect what our brains do in that instant, it can also shape our future behavior," the article states.

In fact, decades of research have found that the more the brain contemplates a behavior, the more likely it is that we will engage in it. Questions make us stop and think and focus solely on what is being asked. They "prompt the brain to contemplate a behavior, which increases the probability that it will be acted upon," the article states. Thus, asking for help through a series of questions is a powerful way to influence physicians you want in your coalition.

At Duke LifePoint Hospital in UP Marquette, Brian Sinotte, CEO, and Dr. David Grant, Chief of Staff, engaged their physicians in a dialogue by hosting a physician retreat and summit in preparation for the board meeting. The physician retreat focused on asking a lot of questions, including:

- ☐ What is working, not working?

- ☐ Why do we exist as an organization?

- ☐ What should be our vision, clinically and business wise?

- ☐ Where are we today on a high performance continuum that includes five stages of forming, struggling, stable, on mission, and high performing?

- ☐ Where do we want to be collectively on this continuum in the next few years?

- ☐ Where are our priorities short term and long term?

- ☐ What are the obstacles to achieve our vision?

- ☐ What do we need to do differently?

- ☐ How do we change our structure, especially MEC to support our vision?

  This meeting took place before a board meeting. The physician inputs were critical in shaping the board strategy. The physician engagement was key in the turn around.

Powerful questions to engage others:

Situate

- ☐ What is your perspective on this issue/matter?

- ☐ On a scale of 1 to 5, where 1 is "I am against it," and 5 is "I am ALL IN," where do you stand?

- ☐ What would it take to get you to a 5?

- ☐ How would you describe the current situation?

- ☐ Is the current situation acceptable to you?

- ☐ What assumptions do you have about this situation/ issue?

- ☐ What is the part you are willing to play to advance this outcome?

- ☐ Do you see an opportunity going forward for us to work together?

- ☐ Do you see a potential better state?

- ☐ Do you see a need to change, shift the way we do it today?

Humanize

- ☐ What is important to you?

- ☐ What do you value the most?

- ☐ If you were the patient, what would you want/expect?

- ☐ If you were the physician, what would you want/ expect?

- ☐ What threats do you see?

- ☐ What opportunities do you see?

- ☐ What concerns you the most?

- ☐ What feelings can you share to help me understand your position?

- ☐ What intrigues you the most about this idea?

Co-Create

- ☐ If there is no limitation, what could be an ideal solution or outcome?

- ☐ What can we do together to combine the best of our thoughts?

- ☐ How can we merge our different ideas?

- ☐ What can we do to build common ground?

- ☐ What can we do to get the best result?

- ☐ What would be a game changer?

- ☐ If you had your choice, what would you do?

- ☐ What can we do to build trust in this situation?

- ☐ What is the desired outcome?

- ☐ How can we create a win-win situation?

- ☐ What questions do you have that might guide us forward?

- ☐ What are we missing?

- ☐ Is there another perspective we are missing?

- ☐ Who else needs to be involved?

- ☐ Where can this plan fail?

Sprint

- ☐ If we would want to try one thing, what would that be?

- ☐ Would you be willing to try one thing for a limited time?

- ☐ If we could implement any solution, what would you go for?

- ☐ What hassle factor is in your daily work that impacts you and your care?

- ☐ If there is one hassle factor that we can remove together what would that be?

- ☐ What if we try this____, would it work?

- ☐ What if we try this ____, would you try it?

Styles Matter

First, let's consider physicians' communication styles. In my work at CTI Physician Leadership Institute, I have spent years helping physicians and administrators learn about their styles and how those help or hinder effectiveness. We use a style assessment, called DiSC, which the physicians take to assess Dominance, Influence, Steadiness and Consciousness tendency. As a result of our work, a study of the 1,583 physicians who took the assessment showed how styles may impact engagement. Of all the assessments taken:

- 24 percent identified as Dominant, which signifies being independent-minded, autonomous, results-oriented, and quick to act to accomplish tasks

- 28 percent identified as Conscientious, which signifies advocating for accuracy, perfection, having high standards, and being uncomfortable making mistakes

- 24 percent identified as Influential, those who are enthusiastic, enjoy engaging with others, and spending time in conversation

- 24 percent identified as Steady, those who are don't like too much change and are dependable and patient

Knowing physicians' styles allows us to adjust the way we communicate with them:

- If you are engaging a physician with a Dominant style, stick to the facts and results

- If you are engaging a physician with an Influence style, spend more time on personal relationships and conversations

- If you are engaging a physician with a Consciousness style, ensure accuracy and high standards

- If you are engaging a physician with a Steadiness style, allow time for them to process the change

Adjusting your communication to the listener style will have a more effective outcome on engagement.

The Way We Communicate Matters

In times of change, it is crucial for a leader to be "hyper-communicating." Use the rule of sixes: communicate the same message six different times, six different ways. One email does not suffice. Physicians are very busy professionals and communicating with them via email is the least effective method. We must be able to quickly outline the vision for the shift in a type of elevator speech that shows the need for the shift and why their engagement is necessary.

This was the strategy Damian (Pat) Alagia III, MD, MBA, CMO of KentuckyOne, utilized to partner and engage his physicians. After assessing the terrain, the overarching factors to disengagement was one of transparency, accountability, inclusion and collaboration.

Physicians want to be included in the conversations and the decisions that affect their profession, their patients, the place they work, and their peers.

Healthcare organizations can no longer afford to separate the clinical, financial, and operational components of the systems; rather, they must learn to integrate each component in the whole system, like the interwoven strands of DNA.

As a physician himself, Alagia had a good idea of what doctors wanted from administrators. And it didn't include a bunch of directives.

"I don't think you ever get engaged through power. I always work from the position that I have to help them understand why a change is important and why it has value to them or their colleagues."

Alagia set out to try to get physicians to co-create with him by forming physician leadership councils that met routinely to discuss various challenging topics such as:

- Wait times in the emergency room
- The implementation of ICD 10
- The Ebola virus outbreak
- The nursing shortage

He also held physician leadership meetings where leaders from the service lines met monthly to focus on transparency, trust, and length of stay. At the end of many of the meetings, physicians were given three action items to enact. Again, this was a way to empower the physicians to co-create together and make them more accountable and engaged, while building trust in the process.

Another step involved working with CTI to help create a physician leadership pathway to provide physician leaders with the "business" tools they would need to work effectively with their non-clinical colleagues.

And using a co-creation step-by-step approach to build trust, Alagia addressed many of the physicians' needs and concerns:

- To follow through on their commitment to communicate with physicians, they created a widely circulated and read bi-monthly newsletter known as *Doc to Doc.* (Step 4, communication and influence)

- To follow through on their commitment to include physicians in the work occurring throughout the system and within their hospitals, they created venues for those physicians who were interested in, but not fully or formally involved with the hospital leadership, to participate in physician leadership councils, clinical leadership councils, weekly 30-minute flash calls, monthly leadership calls, blue-chip quality councils, town hall meetings, and physician leadership forums.

- And finally, to follow through on their commitment to creating a transparent, high-trust, and collaborative environment between physicians and non-clinical administrative colleagues, they made sure to invite key physician leaders to participate in all meetings.

It wasn't as easy as it sounds, Alagia said. Some non-physician administrators hated the idea of involving physicians in decision-making. "Honesty was a huge part of it, and you sometimes had to have difficult, mature conversations. Sometimes, it was horrible."

Every single week, Alagia had calls with physicians to check in and see how things were going. "My job was to go around and continually water or pollinate and make myself available for physician discussions."

He emphasized that being a doctor made his job a bit easier because the physicians tended to respect his ideas and opinions more than those of non-physician leaders. His influence was increasing.

"I think you need to have physician leadership. A nurse can't do some of these things. Some physician needs to be the brand manager. You need a doc."

Over three years, the engagement levels rose by 28%. Not a huge spike, he said, but progress was made and physicians were more engaged. Work continues to raise the engagement scores even higher.

"If you have happy docs, they're going to move things forward. It will carry over to the rest of the team. If you have a grumpy doc, they can bring down the whole team. One or two bad docs can spoil the whole well. That's why achieving high engagement in today's healthcare world is so important."

Consistency of the Message Matters

As you rally more physicians to co-create with you and help you engage others, you need to ensure consistency of the message. One effective way to organize a message, communicate the vision, connect people with deeper purpose, and humanize the conversation is an elevator speech. This tool allows the physicians to customize the message in different ways to connect with the different listeners. The structure of the elevator speech includes 4Ps:

- **Picture:** The **vision** for the change or shift

- **Purpose: Why** this shift matters (from their perspective)

- **Plan:** The action **plan** to achieve the goal

- **Part to play:** What part we'd like them to play and what part we will play

COMMUNICATE THE VISION

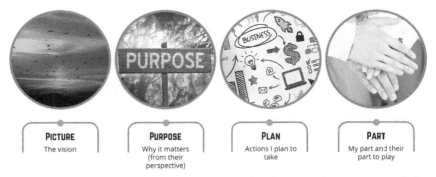

PICTURE	PURPOSE	PLAN	PART
The vision	Why it matters (from their perspective)	Actions I plan to take	My part and their part to play

In our sepsis example, the picture the hospitalists painted for others is that they want to create the safest environment for practicing medicine and caring for patients. The key purposes for applying the sepsis bundle varied from saving lives, reducing length of stay, improving quality, and/or avoiding liability depending on the person they were talking to. Constant communication with all the staff about the importance of the sepsis bundle was applied. Hospitalists, sent emails, featured sepsis bundles in a newsletter including stories of success in saving lives, placed signage in the appropriate departments about sepsis bundles, created a dedicate website, made videos, and held town hall meetings to discuss how the bundles were working.

SEPSIS EXAMPLE

SOURCE	4P	EXAMPLE
Vision	Picture	"I believe (I am committed) we could be the best and safest place for patients and best place to practice."
Why for them	Purpose	I know you care about: • Saving lives • Reducing LOS • Improving quality outcomes • Liability • Giving input
Influence Strategies	Plan	"We've identified sepsis bundle that helped other physicians and organizations achieve this goal and we want to share this bundle with your department."
Source of Disengagement Influence Strategies	Part	I care about you and the team. "I'd like your team's help to learn about the bundle. Can I schedule time with you and your team to discuss.

Listening Matters

It is not sufficient to give your coalition the elevator speech as a tool. It is equally important to provide them with the skills to listen. The statistics are not encouraging. On average, it takes a physician 7 seconds to interrupt a patient or a colleague. That is why it is critical to listen first and seek to understand before being understood.

Frame conversations as dialogues rather than monologues so that people feel that their voices are being heard. Listen to and understand the issues, obstacles, or reasons for disengagement. Use tactics to shift the narrative to reduce fear, ambiguity, and uncertainty, by letting go of being Mr. or Ms. Know-It-All. Increase listening and transparency, share the truth, and spend time on a shared purpose like patient safety and wellbeing.

Don't be afraid to say "I don't know." Be empathetic, compassionate, and willing to walk away as sometimes; it may not be the right time to engage the physician.

Dealing with the Drama and the Brutal Facts

At a certain point along the journey, as you situate and assess the terrain and the level of engagement, humanize the issue, invite others to co-create with you, and listen and have the conversations, you will get to a point, as a physician or as a leader, where you will have to deal with the brutal fact that there are physicians who will not engage with you, your initiative, or your organization. This is a moment of leadership, a moment that requires courage to deal with the brutal facts and drama. By now, you may have heard all the excuses or observed all the behaviors of disengagement. The questions you have to ask yourself as a leader are:

1. Does it matter if they are not engaged? Are they critical to success?

2. Can I accept the fact that not every physician needs to be engaged?

3. Are they a threat if they are actively disengaged or passively aggressive?

4. What shall I do about it?

5. Will I stop parenting and start treating them as professionals? Can I hold them accountable?

6. Do I need to have a crucial, courageous conversation?

In his book "From Good to Great," Jim Collins called this the Stockdale Paradox, after Jim Stockdale, the most senior

United States Navy Vice Admiral and aviator in the Vietnam War. Stockdale was held captive in Hanoi, North Vietnam for more than seven years and was awarded the Medal of Honor. "The Stockdale Paradox is a signature of all those who create greatness, be it leading their own lives or in leading others. It didn't matter how bleak the situation or how stultifying their mediocrity; they all maintained unwavering faith that they would not just survive, but prevail as a great company. And yet, at the same time, they became relentlessly disciplined at confronting the most brutal facts of their current reality."

The Stockdale Paradox is to "retain the faith that you will prevail in the end, regardless of difficulties, and, at the same time, confront the most brutal facts of your current reality, whatever they may be."

Your journey is almost complete. The level of engagement is rising. Engagement is happening. Now, there's just one more leg of the trip to complete. It is about taking incremental steps one sprint at a time.

Summary of Actions – CONVERSE

- ☐ Everything exists in language

- ☐ Trust and engagement are results of one conversation at a time

- ☐ Ensure consistency of the message

- ☐ Use Elevator Speech 4P

  - o **Picture**: The **vision** for the change or shift

  - o **Purpose**: **Why** this shift matters (from their perspective)

  - o **Plan**: The action **plan** to achieve the goal

  - o **Part to play**: What part we'd like them to play and what part we will play

- ☐ Style matters

  - o Customize the message to the physician's communication style

  - o If you are engaging a physician with a Dominant style, stick to the facts and results

  - o If you are engaging a physician with an Influence style, spend more time on personal relationships and conversations

  - o If you are engaging a physician with a Consciousness style, ensure accuracy and high standards

  - o If you are engaging a physician with a Steadiness style, allow time for them to process the change

- ☐ Listening matters – let other people do a great deal of the talking

- ☐ Deal with the drama and brutal facts

Step 5: Sprint

The journey of a thousand miles, starts with the first small step.

-Tao

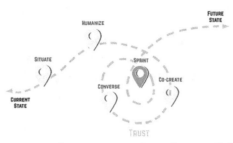

"Don't look for moon shot approaches. Instead focus on hitting singles and doubles every time at bat." An advice from Ron Paulus, MD, President and CEO at Mission Health.

In design thinking, the critical step after ideation is to prototype and test ideas, get feedback, and adjust as necessary. I call this step "Sprint." In this whole process, what matters most is trust. Engaging physicians requires small acts of building trust and "Sprint." The tendency to send survey after survey to assess and measure engagement is looked at as another metric and rarely adds to the trust account. That is why building trust is foundational.

Here are examples of Sprints (BE, KNOW, and DO) that build trust:

1. BE:

    1. Be open to other people's ideas and points of view.

    2. Regulate your emotions, and separate the issue from the emotions.

    3. Never criticize someone in public. Praise in public, coach in private.

4. Model the expected change. Be the change you'd like to see in others.

5. Be venerable. Be willing to admit a mistake you may have made.

6. Be humble. Be willing to say, "I don't know." You don't have to be the smartest person in the room.

7. Be honest and transparent: Share the data and the facts, and tell people where they stand. People make up their own story when they lack information. Tell the truth even when it hurts.

8. Smile and wave! Make someone's day!

2. KNOW

   1. Being present in the clinic, the OR, etc. Being present sends a signal that we are in this together.

   2. Get to know physicians as human beings first. Invite a physician to breakfast or a cup of coffee to check in without having any other agenda.

   3. Allow time for small talk with others, even if you don't believe in it. You will be amazed what you learn.

   4. Provide timely feedback.

   5. Empathy. See what they see every day.

3. DO

   1. Identify a hassle factor that is impacting your physicians in a specific area or unit. You can use the free Hassle Factor IndexTM (HFI) survey online at www.CTIleadership.com.

2. Ask people to weigh-in on the hassle factor and voice their opinions on how it impacts their practice. Allow them to express their frustration, anger, and discontent when appropriate so you can move into discussing potential solutions.

3. Ask physicians to work with you and others on identifying improvement ideas to remove or minimize the hassle factor.

4. Create psychological safety. Create an environment where physicians have confidence that, if they speak up, they will not be shamed, embarrassed, rejected, or punished

5. Hold listening sessions. Make time to listen to your physicians, and truly listen without any filters and biases.

6. Focus on small gains instead of boiling the ocean. Don't take on huge projects or talk to too many people at the same time; focus on small tests of change (focusing on winnable battles).

7. Try-storm instead of brainstorm ideas. Be in continuous innovation and trial of new ideas or improvement. Have the courage to try things for one day or one week. Try-storming builds momentum and energy.

8. Daily stand up huddle. Host a daily stand up huddle with your team or a coalition of physicians you are co-creating with. This is a short meeting while standing up (so it does not have to run for an hour). The agenda is simple:

   - What worked well yesterday?

   - Acknowledge someone on the team for a job well done.

- Read a customer comment or feedback (positive or negative).

- What did not go well? Why?

- What do need to do different today to address and correct?

- What did we try-storm yesterday? Did it work? Or not? Why not? What do we need to adjust?

- What is our try-storming improvement idea today?

9. Have small conversations of encouragement with the coalition as they go about their work engaging the silent majority.

10. Celebrate small wins like a decline in sepsis – even just a slight decline.

11. Personally congratulate the physicians who successfully engage in your mission.

12. Share the WHY: Why are we having a conversation? Why is engagement necessary? Remember, engagement is contextual. Without background information, physicians create their own narratives often leading to fear and uncertainty. Providing context moves physicians from uncertainty to understanding.

13. Focus on the patient, when conversing with your peers by agreeing on ways to provide better care and savings lives.

14. Use logical reasoning, expertise, and/or compelling facts that illustrate the need.

15. Identify and remove hassle factors that make adoption difficult.

16. Provide examples of similar situations and successful outcomes.

17. Make others feel valued by involving them in decision making and giving them recognition.

18. Call an initiative, or a project, a "shift" as opposed to a "change".

19. Talk about doing the right thing for the patient as opposed to "compliance."

20. Share reliable performance data as evidence for the shift.

21. Focus on positive results, not bad outcomes.

22. Illustrate what best practices look like.

23. Celebrate when people identify failures, especially red on a score card. Allen Mullaly, Previous CEO of Ford Motor and Boeing, used to stand up and clap when someone identified a red on a score card. Allen said, "I would rather have people identify failures so we can deal with them together instead of managing lies."

24. Provide regular feedback on the progress being made.

25. Establish processes, policies, and norms to support and enable the change, including incentives, rewards, and recognition.

26. Use digital tools to open dialogue with your physicians (Waggl tool for example)

I have seen Sprint being used effectively at Mission Health. In Asheville, North Carolina, the state's sixth-largest health system and has been recognized as one of the nation's Top 15 Health Systems in five of six years from 2012 to 2017 by Truven Health Analytics/IBM Watson (formerly Thomson Reuters). Dr. Ron Paulus, President and CEO of Mission Health, explains:

"First, we focus on priorities on a weekly basis with [a program known as] Standout. Standout is based on Marcus Buckingham's work of assessing an individual's strengths and finding his or her edge using a strengths-based engagement and performance management system. Ensuring ongoing dialogue and dedication to short-term actions allows the team to concentrate on the business at hand.

"Second, on a regular basis, we look at our long-term strategies and we adjust our actions and priorities as needed.

"At Mission, we manage change by hardwiring our focus into our tasks and working together collaboratively every single week."

Another level of engagement is through service line report-out meetings. These are meetings with key service-line leaders and their dyad partners, Paulus said. The conversations are grounded in evidence, actual performance, and data—not random opinions.

"These meetings are a great model of active engagement and leadership and provide an excellent format and structure to discuss successes, failures, and, most importantly, the need for help."

Having people in the right positions is important, too. "We were very intentional in creating new chief roles (in between a vice president and a senior vice president). We mentor and develop the chief cohort on an ongoing basis. In creating a chief role, we may add to a leader's responsibilities an uncommon area—say parking for the chief quality officer—to expose that leader to areas they would not have access to normally.

Summary of Actions – SPRINT

- ☐ The journey of a thousand miles, starts with the first small step

- ☐ One sprint and conversation at a time would lead to trust and engagement

- ☐ Use BE, KNOW, DO sprints to deepen trust and engagement

- ☐ Be open, humble, honest, and visible

- ☐ Get to know physicians as human beings; empathize and see the world from their perspective. Small talks are a good thing.

- ☐ Try-storm new ideas

- ☐ Simply have the conversation

- ☐ Create psychological safety where people are open to expressing their thoughts and concerns without fear of consequences.

- ☐ Hold listening sessions

- ☐ Identify hassle factors and engage others to remove them

- ☐ Smile, wave, and make someone's day!

Outcomes

At Catholic Health Initiative, by focusing on Sepsis, the hospital medicine physicians and leaders were able to accomplish the following annual results:

- Saved 2,299 lives

- Reduced excess days by 17,385

- Prevented 3,716 readmissions

- Significant improvements in "culture of ownership"

- Clinical standards; documentation standards

In addition, the hospitalists that participated in the CHI Physician Leadership Fellowship, reported the following improvement:

- 64% improvement in the ability to lead others more effectively.

- 65% improvement in the ability to work more effectively in teams.

- 31% improvement in the ability to solve problems more effectively.

- 73% improvement in the ability to communicate with and influence others.

- 83% improvement in the ability to deal more effectively with difficult issues.

- 44% improvement in the ability to work well with their clinical/admin teams.

- 57% improvement in the ability to work well with the executive team.

- 29% improvement in the level of commitment to and active engagement in ensuring the organization's success.

- 30% improvement in the loyalty to the organization.

- 22% improvement in the willingness to serve in a leadership capacity within the organization.

At Lee Health, Dr. Scott Nygaard is now leveraging the return on his investment in developing and engaging his physicians. The physicians that have gone through structured fellowship and were engaged in clinical and operational project work reported improvement in their willingness to engage, engagement by their staff, willingness to take on leadership roles, and increased satisfaction and loyalty to the organization (ALL IN). The following are the **overall average improvements** after participating in the Lee Health Physician Leadership Fellowship:

- **45% improvement** in the ability **to collaborate in teams.**

- **42% improvement** in the ability **to solve problems innovatively.**

- **54% improvement** in the ability **to communicate and influence.**

- **41% improvement** in the ability **to build relationships with others.**

- **70% improvement** in the ability **to deal with difficult issues/conversations.**

- **56% improvement** in the ability **to accept their role as a leader.**

- **58% improvement** in the ability **to work with the executive team.**

- **45% improvement** in the **willingness to be engaged in the organization.**

- **41% improvement** in their **staff's level of engagement.**

- **44% improvement** in the **willingness to serve in a leadership capacity.**

- **15% improvement** in the **loyalty to the organization.**

- **28% improvement** in the **level of their work satisfaction.**

- **38% improvement** in the **level of their team's moral/work satisfaction.**

Similarly, at Mission Health, Dr. Ron Paulus, is leveraging the return on his investment in developing and engaging his physicians. The physicians that have gone through structured fellowship and were engaged in clinical and operational project work reported improvement in their willingness to engage, engagement by their staff, willingness to take on leadership roles, and increased satisfaction. The following are the **overall average improvements** after participating in the Mission Health Clinician Leadership Fellowship:

- **25% improvement** in the ability **to collaborate in teams.**

- **25% improvement** in the ability **to solve problems innovatively.**

- **61% improvement** in the ability **to communicate and influence.**

- **24% improvement** in the ability **to build relationships with others.**

- **55% improvement** in the ability **to deal with difficult issues/conversations.**

- **48% improvement** in the ability **to accept their role as a leader.**

- **32% improvement** in the ability **to work with their clinical/admin teams.**

- **30% improvement** in the ability **to work with the executive team.**

- **36% improvement** in the **willingness to be engaged in the organization.**

- **52% improvement** in their **staff's level of engagement.**

- **30% improvement** in the **willingness to serve in a leadership capacity.**

- **17% improvement** in the **loyalty to the organization.**

Similarly, at Duke LifePoint Marquette, Brian Sinotte, CEO, is leveraging the return on his organization investment in developing and engaging his physicians. The physicians reported improvement in their willingness to engage, loyalty to the organization, engagement by their staff, willingness to take on leadership roles, and increased satisfaction.

The participants reported the following **overall average improvements** after participating in the Physician Leadership Fellowship at Marquette:

- **33% improvement** in the ability **to collaborate in teams.**

- **20% improvement** in the ability **to solve problems innovatively.**

- **92% improvement** in the ability **to communicate and influence.**

- **60% improvement** in the ability **to build relationships with others.**

- **78% improvement** in the ability **to deal with difficult issues/conversations.**

- **58% improvement** in the ability **to accept their role as a leader.**

- **39% improvement** in the ability **to work with their clinical/admin teams.**

- **61% improvement** in the ability **to work with the executive team.**

- **61% improvement** in the **willingness to be engaged in the organization.**

- **41% improvement** in their **staff's level of engagement.**

- **40% improvement** in the **willingness to serve in a leadership capacity.**

- **64% improvement** in the **loyalty to the organization.**

- **41% improvement** in the **level of their work satisfaction.**

- **64% improvement** in the **level of their team's moral/work satisfaction.**

Finally, at The Iowa Clinic, Ed Brown, CEO, is leveraging the return on his investment in on-boarding physicians. His new physicians reported improvement in their willingness to engage, loyalty to the organization, commitment to quality and safety, willingness to take on leadership roles, and increased satisfaction in their decision to join the Clinic. The following are the **overall average ratings** after participating in the Iowa Clinic Physician On-Boarding Academy:

- **Integrating into TIC has accelerated:** 75%

- **Feeling supported by TIC:** 98%

- **Establishing a network of support among new and current physicians and staff:** 88%

- **Understanding of the importance of the patient experience has improved:** 87%

- **Being able to act as a change agent:** 80%

- **Working with clinical and administrative team members has improved:** 75%

- **Commitment to/engagement in ensuring TIC's success has increased:** 87%

- **Loyalty to TIC increased:** 80%

- **Willingness to serve in a leadership capacity at TIC has increased:** 80%

- **Confidence in the fact that I made the decision to join TIC has increased:** 90%

These results show the averages while individual improvements were more than 10 times the averages. This is the power of co-creation: the return of investment in physicians and the value of partnering with physicians. Loyalty, engagement in quality and safety, and willingness to serve in leadership capacity are great measures of success. They demonstrate that the Engagement Roadmap works and works well. Now it is your turn to achieve similar return on investment.

Summary

So having read this far and pondered the success stories, it's time for you to ask yourself the following questions: "Where does my organization or team land on the engagement continuum? Do we have a high-performing healthcare team of physicians and other medical staff who are ALL-IN and constantly work together to solve problems, interact professionally, and strive to provide the absolutely best and safest patient care? Do we have a group of motivated and energized team members and leaders who go above and beyond, encourage and embrace other team members to achieve ever-higher goals, and take on new challenges?"

If that sounds like your organization, congratulations! Yours is among an elite group of highly engaged workplaces. Or, does your organization lie at the other end of the spectrum, with physicians and other staff who are ALL OUT, plodding through each day and simply doing the absolute minimum? Do they grumble about the schedule, the workload, and sometimes squabble among themselves? Is your staff infected with a large group of "no-joes" who resist nearly every new idea or best practice?

We certainly hope you're not operating under those conditions.

More than likely, your organization—like most—falls somewhere in between the two extremes. And it also may be likely that you aren't too sure what the level of engagement is in your organization because you haven't taken the time to measure, study, understand, and improve it.

Don't worry, you're not alone. We believe a majority of healthcare organizations have not made physician engagement a top priority. It's time then for a road trip, and we're not talking about a quick jaunt across town. We're talking about a long journey—in fact, a never-ending journey— that will propel your organization to new heights of engagement, cooperation, and accomplishments.

Start by being contextual. Situate yourself and map the terrain. Figure out where your physicians stand, and determine where to concentrate your efforts. Humanize the issue or conversation by aligning your engagement effort to a relevant purpose that will resound with the physicians and staff. In other words, target something that touches their values and concerns.

Next, build a coalition of physicians that will co-create with you and eventually influence others, particularly the silent majority, to embrace the initiative and join the movement. Make sure you invest in them and give them the skills and tools to be more effective at influencing and engaging others. Finally, build trust one conversation at a time and one sprint at a time. As you experience the first successes and engagement beginning to blossom in your organization, anchor it in the culture and make it the norm, not the exception.

Yes, it's going to be a long journey that is difficult and sometimes frustrating. Yes, you'll sometimes question whether this road trip holds value. But, ultimately, when you again map the terrain in the future and find physicians engaged and all in with you along the journey, you'll know that the trip was worth it.

Ultimately, you will be successful by rethinking engagement as being two-way commitment, by partnering with your physicians, by humanizing the issue and inviting others to co-create with us. You will be successful by reducing the stress of big initiatives by focusing on one conversation at the time, and by doing as many sprints which build trust and, eventually, engagement.

Imagine a world of healthcare where every physician is engaged, emotionally connected, and contributing to his or her full intellectual capacity. A world where every physician is ALL-IN and happier because he or she feels heard. A world where everyone sees his or her self as an active team member and a collaborative leader.

This is possible. It's not an imaginary nirvana. The shared roadmap to engagement will help you chart the course. I've seen it work, and I am confident it will work for you. It will take a shift in how you see engagement. Engagement is not a metric; it is a reciprocal commitment that we make to each other as professionals. It is a leadership act. It starts with you, the leader, but, does not end with you. The physicians have to make a choice to engage and be ALL IN or not.

Engagement is about humanizing the issue or challenge. It is about co-creating solutions with your physicians. It is achieved one conversation at a time, a conversation that inspires trust.

Time to hit the road.

Enjoy your journey.

Giving Thanks

Writing this book was more rewarding than I could have ever imagined. None of this would have been possible without the expertise and knowledge shared by so many wonderful friends and colleagues.

I'd like to thank Ron Paulus, Pat Alagia, Alan Rosenstein, William Cors, Scott Nygaard, Brian Sinotte, William Martin, Jeff Moreadith, Michael Hein, Willie Lawrence, Gary Ridge, Joe Cozzolino, Grace Terrell, Joann Farrell Quinn, Dan Kollmorgen, and Ed Brown for their keen insight and ongoing commitment to physician leadership and engagement. It is because of their exquisite leadership and sharing of experiences that I was able to create and share this engagement road map with you all.

My deep gratitude to Randy Haffner for his willingness to share the personal story of his daughter, Bailey, and inspiring all of us to humanize our conversation and engage others as human beings and not human doings.

A very special thanks to Dr. Marshall Goldsmith and my fellow MG100 coaches. The friendships and comradery that I have discovered through my involvement in Dr. Marshall Goldsmith's Pay It Forward project are immeasurably rewarding. A big "Thank You" to Chester Elton and Ayse Birsel for their support and encouragement.

My great appreciation to everyone on our CTI team with whom I have the benefit of serving alongside each and every day! You inspire me to dream big and continue to grow! Mallory, your attention to details is always invaluable.

Special thanks and gratitude for Bill Stagier for his help and support on this book.

Finally, to my wife Rana, thank you for your unending encouragement, support, vision and contribution that truly are the reasons this book became a reality.

References and Resources

ABIM Foundation videos, June 2012, Finding Joy in Primary Care.

http://abimfoundation.org/videos

Accessed 12/28/2017

Agency for Healthcare Research and Quality.

https://www.ahrq.gov/professionals/clinicians-providers/ahrq-works/burnout/index.html

Accessed 12/26/2017

Behreini, S. Employee Engagement is More Important Than the Customer

https://www.entrepreneur.com/article/247797

October 15, 2015

Accessed 2/26/2018

Bill Hudec, Advisory Board, "The 12 statements that define your physicians' engagement," June 25, 2015.

https://www.advisory.com/research/medical-group-strategy-council/practice-notes/2015/june/who-is-to-blame-for-physician-burnout

Burger, J and Sutton, L. *How Employee Engagement Can Improve a Hospital's Health*

http://www.gallup.com/businessjournal/168149/employee-engagement-improve-hospital-health.aspx

Accessed 2/27/2018

Infographic: The Importance of Employee Engagement NBRI

https://www.nbrii.com/blog/infographic/

Accessed 2/26/2018

Custominsight

https://www.custominsight.com/

Accessed 2/26/2018

Drummund, Dike, MD, blog post on The Happy MD website.

https://www.thehappymd.com/blog/bid/295048/physician-burnout-why-its-not-a-fair-fight

Accessed 12/26/2017

Glaser, Judith E. Conversational Intelligence: How Great Leaders Build Trust and Get Extraordinary Results. Taylor and Francis. Kindle Edition.

Hoffeld, D. "Want to Know What Your Brain Does When It Hears a Question?"

https://www.fastcompany.com/3068341/want-to-know-what-your-brain-does-when-it-hears-a-question

Accessed 3/1/2018

Jim Collins. Good to Great. Harper Business, 2001

Johnson, C. Bad Blood: Doctor-Nurse Behavior Problems Impact Patient Care. Tampa, FL, American College of Physician Executives, PEJ, November-December 2009.

Kruse, K. What is Employee Engagement?, Forbes, June 22, 2012.

http://www.forbes.com/sites/kevinkruse/2012/06/22/employee-engagement-what-and-why/#790262454629

Accessed 2/26/2018

O'byrne, T. History of Employee Engagement—From Satisfaction to Sustainability

http://www.hrzone.com/engage/employees/history-of-employee-engagement-from-satisfaction-to-sustainability

Accessed 2/26/2018

Pink, D. H. (2012). *Drive: the surprising truth about what motivates us.* New York, NY: Riverhead Books.

Shanafelt TD, Hasan O, Dyrbye LN, Sinsky C, Satele D, and others. (2015) Changes in Burnout and Satisfaction with Work-Life Blanace and the General U.S. Working Population Between 2011-2014. Mayo Clin Proc 90(12).

Sherwood, R. *Employee Engagement Drive Health Care Quality and Financial Returns*

https://hbr.org/2013/10/employee-engagement-drives-health-care-quality-and-financial-returns

Accessed 2/27/2018

SHRM: Employee Engagement, Your Competitive Advantage https://www.shrm.org/ResourcesAndTools/business-solutions/Documents/Engagement%20Briefing-FINAL.pdf

Accessed 2/26/2018

Sinah, Pranay, MD, How to find joy in practicing medicine, KevinMD blog post, 9/18/2017.

https://www.kevinmd.com/blog/2017/09/find-joy-practicing-medicine.html

Accessed 12/28/2017

"The Engagement Gap: Physicians Aren't As Engaged as Executives Think."

https://www.jacksonphysiciansearch.com/wp-content/uploads/2016/09/resource-1-smaller.pdf

Ton, Z and Kalloch, S. How 4 Retailers Became the "Best Places to Work."

https://hbr.org/2017/01/how-4-retailers-became-best-places-to-work

Accessed 2/27/2018

Vorhauser-Smith, S. *How the Best Places to Work are Nailing Employee Engagement*

http://www.forbes.com/sites/sylviavorhausersmith/2013/08/14/how-the-best-places-to-work-are-nailing-employee-engagement/#6284d06938aa

Accessed 2/27/2018

Want to Increase Hospital Revenues? Engage Your Physicians. When doctors are frustrated, patient care and hospital revenues suffer. Here's how to boost physicians' engagement -- and the bottom line. BY JEFF BURGER AND ANDREW GIGER

https://news.gallup.com/businessjournal/170786/increase-hospital-revenues-engage-physicians.aspx

Sample Engagement Roadmap

ENGAGEMENT MAP

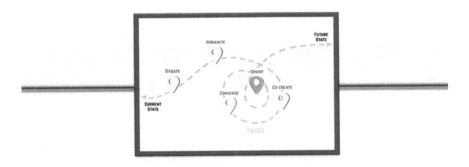

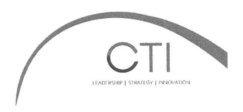

SITUATE (Map the Terrain)			
Name of Individual or Group	**Engagement Level** 1-----2-----3-----4-----5 Checked Out Aligned All In		**How Critical** 1---2---3---4---5 Low Med High
	CURRENT	DESIRED	
SAMPLE: Hospital Medicine Group	2	4	4
1.			
2.			
3.			
4.			
5.			
6.			
7.			
8.			
9.			
10.			

HUMANIZE (Assess the Terrain)		
Selected Individual or Group (Critical, Low Engagement):	**Current Behaviors**	**Optimal Behaviors**

Their Interests, Concerns & Assumptions	*Their* Motivators	
	What **OPPORTUNITIES** are likely to arise if the change IS made?	What **THREATS** may arise if the change IS NOT made?

CTI

CO-CREATE (Engage a Coalition)	
All In and Engaged Groups	**How They Can Help Champion the Effort and Engage Others**

CONVERSE			
Personalized Narrative (Tailored to Individual Concerns)			
Picture (Vision)	**Purpose** (Why it Matters)	**Plan** (Proposed Solutions)	**Part to Play** (Their part & Our Part)

SPRINT	
Influence Actions	**Early Wins**

COMMITMENTS

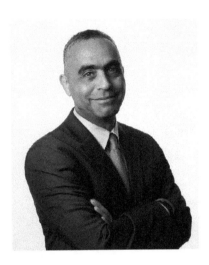

Mo Kasti is a distinguished author, coach, entrepreneur, speaker, strategy advisor and family man. His passion is to save lives by helping executives and clinical leaders elevate their thinking in times of transformation and capitalize on emerging innovation opportunities.

Mo is the author of the international best-selling book, "Physician Leadership," The RX to Healthcare Transformation. He is the CEO and founder of the nationally recognized Physician Leadership Institute (PLI) dedicated to accelerating healthcare transformation through leadership and innovation. He is one of the top MG100 Coaches, Dr. Marshall Goldsmith's Pay It Forward project.

Mo's previous roles include Chief Transformation Officer and Chief Operating Officer (COO) for USF Health and has held successful leadership roles with General Electric Healthcare (NYSE: GE).

Mo lives in Tampa, Florida with his wife and two sons. His blog is found at: www.mokasti.com and he can be reached at: mkasti@ctileadership.com